Comprehensive arthroscopic examination of the knee

Comprehensive arthroscopic examination of the knee

LANNY L. JOHNSON, M.D.

Clinical Associate Professor of Surgery
College of Human Medicine
Michigan State University
East Lansing, Michigan

with 161 illustrations, including 94 in full color

THE C. V. MOSBY COMPANY

Saint Louis   1977

The C. V. Mosby Company
11830 Westline Industrial Drive, St. Louis, Missouri 63141

Library of Congress Cataloging in Publication Data

Johnson, Lanny L
    Comprehensive arthroscopic examination of
the knee.

    Includes bibliographical references and index.
    1. Knee—Examination. 2. Arthroscopy. I. Title.
[DNLM: 1. Knee joint. 2. Joint diseases—
Diagnosis. 3. Endoscopy. WE870 J67c]
RD561.J63   617'.582   77-21646
ISBN 0-8016-2534-3

TS/U/B 9 8 7 6 5 4 3 2 1

Preface

Arthroscopy is a dynamic, colorful, and exciting experience for the physician. It is best appreciated by performing the procedure. A one-on-one method of teaching is ideal, but because of time and logistics, it is just not possible. The second-best method of experiencing arthroscopy or learning the technique is by movie photography or television.

In this book, an attempt has been made to duplicate the experience of arthroscopy by logos, photographic selection, diagrams, and design. The color illustrations were carefully chosen to be representative rather than comprehensive.

This book is written for the physician who desires the practical details necessary to successfully accomplish a complete inspection of the knee joint. A description of technical details is necessarily labored. The role of the assistant is included to help the inexperienced arthroscopist.

The physician who perseveres will be rewarded with increased knowledge from arthroscopy. The patient will benefit in better diagnostic judgments and therapeutic designs.

I acknowledge and am exceedingly grateful to my assistant, Mrs. Ruth L. Becker, LPN, who has contributed many of the details of this technique. Her contribution has been recognized by the many visiting physicians as being the most essential ingredient in my ability to perform arthroscopy so easily. I agree.

I appreciate the encouragement I received from Dr. David Shneider, who has been able to completely duplicate this technique with great facility and finesse. Using these methods, he has made observations that have added to my understanding.

Gloria Aveiro typed manuscript and revisions at times undoubtedly inconvenient for her; for this I am grateful. For most of the black-and-white photographs, I thank Tom A. Cannel.

Most of all I appreciate Mary Ann, my wife, and our daughters, Charlotte Ann and Autumn Lynn, who have been faithful in many adventures, including this book.

P.T.L.

Lanny L. Johnson, M.D.

Contents

Comprehensive arthroscopic examination of the knee

Chapter 1

Development

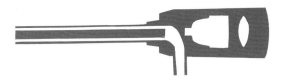

As with any development, the comprehensive arthroscopic examination of the knee evolved from the contributions of pioneers in the field of arthroscopy. Those of Casscells,[1] Jackson,[3,4] and Watanabe[9] are well known. Most orthopedists are well versed in the traditional technique, that is, the use of the large-diameter endoscope, such as a Watanabe No. 21, through which only the anterior compartments of the joint can be viewed. An elaborate irrigation system is used, and the procedure is carried out with the patient under general anesthesia.

Watanabe[10] has stated that the No. 24 arthroscope can be used in the knee joint, although such use is under investigation, but it is not suitable for general diagnostic purposes in this area. McGinty[7] and O'Connor[8] have adapted more modern endoscopes to the classic method.

Eikelaar[2] presents an excellent comprehensive historical review of arthroscopy. No attempt is made to duplicate his effort here; rather, I will detail the development of small-diameter arthroscopes and my experience with them.

INSTRUMENTATION

In 1970 the first self-focusing arthroscope was developed through the joint efforts of the Nippon Sheet Glass Company and the Department of Orthopaedic Surgery of Tokyo Teishin Hospital. This scope, 1.7 mm in diameter, was utilized through a cannula having an outside diameter of 2 mm and provided a direct view of 37° in saline. It was introduced in North America in January 1972 by Mr. Leonard J. Bonnell. To my knowledge, it was first used for arthroscopy by Drs. Clement Sledge and J. Drennen Lowell at the Robert Brigham Hospital, Boston, Massachusetts.

After viewing a single procedure, Mr. Harold L. Neuman assessed the uses of and requirements for such a small-diameter endoscope. The original Watanabe No. 24 arthroscope was redesigned in four ways. The diameter of the endoscope was increased from 1.7 to 2.2 mm, which improved the illumination by a factor of

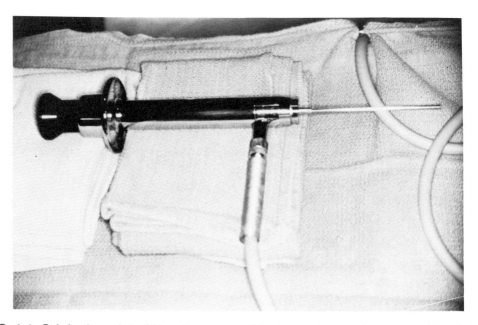

FIG. 1-1. Original model of Needlescope, with three-piece arthroscope. Headpiece screwed onto stainless steel handle. There was a barrier between handle and eyepiece to prevent contamination of the hand by the arthroscopist's head. Eyepiece was inserted manually by a separate maneuver. Disadvantage of this system was that it allowed collection of small dust particles, which when magnified obscured viewing.

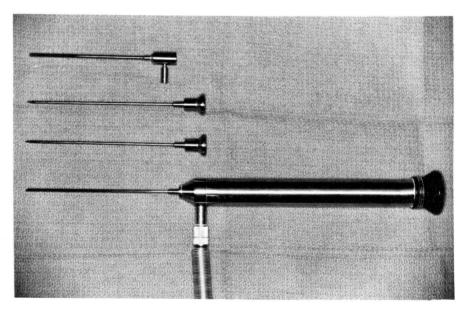

FIG. 1-2. Third model of Needlescope is a closed system with a viewing angle of approximately 70° in saline. Endoscope shown here is 2.2 mm in outside diameter. Cannula, which is superior, has an outside sheath of 2.6 mm in diameter. Sharp and blunt trocars accompany system.

four and resulted in a more rugged assembly. The design was changed to allow for a detachable light guide to improve handling and ease of sterilization. The eyepiece, which required manual focusing, was changed to a fixed-focus lens to reduce confusion and contamination during the procedure. A long lightweight handle was designed for manipulation of the lens so that the physician's head and eye were away from the sterile field and his glove was protected from becoming contaminated.

This three-piece instrument, the Needlescope, was available for marketing in the fall of 1972 (Fig. 1-1). It had a fore-oblique view of 47° in saline, but was rejected by many arthroscopists because of its fragility, low illumination, and reduced optical clarity as compared with existing large-diameter endoscopes of different construction. Additionally, the cover lens in the interior was vulnerable to the collection of small dirt particles, which when magnified obscured the view. Therefore, the second model of the Needlescope was developed with a nitrogen-sealed optical system, which gave consistently satisfactory viewing.

By June 1976 the third model of the Needlescope was being tested. It was enhanced by optical design of the terminal lens to increase its field of view in saline to 70°. Another modification improved the light illumination capacity by at least two f-stops. There now was a small-diameter endoscope with an angle of visualization equal to that of the largest scope and with a facility to document with optical clarity that was competitive with the largest diameter arthroscopes (Fig. 1-2).

TECHNIQUE
First arthroscopy with local anesthetic

The capacity to view the anterior chambers of the knee joint arthroscopically held a great attraction. However, the length of the procedure, the size of the incision including suture closure, and the use of general anesthetic detracted from its practical application. It was difficult to make a strong argument for an arthroscopic examination when the concensus was that the knee, including its anterior chambers, could be better visualized by arthrotomy in less time and with a less elaborate surgical setup than with a large-diameter endoscope.

I had not been attracted to the Watanabe technique because of the above-mentioned objections. However, on October 30, 1972, without having witnessed any arthroscopies, I examined an athlete who had undergone knee surgery but had exacerbation of knee problems with an effusion. The arthroscopic procedure was carried out with the patient under local anesthesia and with tourniquet control. The intra-articular structures were visualized, and cleansing of the joint was possible. A diagnosis of degenerative arthritis with loose bodies was established.

I was excited about the ease with which this examination was accomplished and the observations that could be made. My enthusiasm was not shared by others, however; in fact, the endoscope manufacturer doubted the success of the procedure on the basis of letters received from established arthroscopists. Although limitations in technique and understanding of the arthroscopic image were recognized, I was encouraged to offer this procedure to other patients with knee problems. Ten such arthroscopies were performed in the following month. Experience established confidence and the ability to visualize the interior compartments of the knee joint by arthroscopy with local anesthetic.

A Needlescope was purchased on the basis of satisfaction with my first arthroscopic experience. By the time the instrument arrived, the quality of the lens had been improved. Originally, the lens was processed with a thalium salt ionizing procedure. In the interval, this was changed to use cesium. Resolution was improved by a factor of 10, further enhancing the diagnostic capacity.

Because the early model of the Needlescope lacked in optical quality and had a limitation in angle of view (47° inclined), it was necessary to compensate technically. The concepts of "pistoning," or moving in and out with the endoscope, and scanning back and forth were introduced. These techniques are applicable to and commonly used with any endoscope but are essential with the Needlescope. In arthroscopy, as in surgery, one learns to work from known to unknown. When the surgeon is unsure of an anatomic relationship, he goes back to areas of known structure. In the knee the landmark of most common orientation is the tangential view of the femoral condyle, or the "horizon" of the femoral condyle. The horizon is followed by moving from one compartment to the other for orientation during inspection of the knee joint.

By 1973, arguments against the traditional arthroscopic technique were being resolved. The technique was modified to eliminate the use of general anesthetic, prolonged time needed to perform the technique, incision with suture, and the elaborate water-drainage system. With the patient under local anesthesia, it was possible to visualize the interior of the knee joint better through a 2-mm skin puncture than by the largest arthrotomy short of disarticulation.

In September 1973, Diagnostic Arthroscopy of the Knee[5] was presented at the International Congress. This paper reviewed the first 100 arthroscopies, many of them performed with the patient under local anesthesia, and showed some of the early photographic documentation on slides.

Clinical value of arthroscopy

The clinical value of arthroscopy was now established. Because it could be performed with patients under local anesthesia, they could be placed in two clinical categories. The first group included those patients for whom diagnosis could not be well established by history, physical or x-ray examination, or arthrography and in whom findings were insufficient to warrant surgical exploration under general anesthesia. Arthroscopy with local anesthetic was recommended.

The second group comprised those patients who showed clear-cut evidence of intra-articular abnormality or ligamentous injury. Arthroscopy was performed immediately preceeding an anticipated arthrotomy. The procedure substantiated that many lesions missed by unicompartmental arthrotomy were visualized by arthroscopy. Arthroscopic examination prior to arthrotomy lends confidence in that complete examination. In many cases the preoperative diagnosis was either erroneous or incomplete. Additionally, the surgical design was frequently modified after arthroscopy.

Posteromedial puncture routine

During the first year of arthroscopic experience, it was recognized that inspection of the anterior compartments and the suprapatellar pouch was inadequate. Although it was possible to document abnormalities under the meniscus, even in the areas of the coronary ligament, diagnoses of posterior tears of the medial meniscus were going unrecognized. Inspection of the posteromedial compartment was initiated on every patient in whom anterior examination showed that compartment to be normal. It was not surprising to find that a number of these patients had meniscal tears in the posterior compartment or loose bodies not visible from the front. It was also recognized that the posterior cruciate ligament was easily visualized in many patients from the posteromedial approach. Thus this approach became part of the routine examination.

Posterolateral puncture routine

Many attempts were made to view the knee posterolaterally. Even from an anterolateral approach, it is impossible to completely visualize the posterolateral compartment except in patients with marked ligamentous laxity. From that view the popliteus tendon can be seen at its origin on the lateral femoral condyle, but the mass of the meniscus and the tendon will block the view into the sulcus. Various attempts had been made from different angles to achieve access to that space. In September 1975 it was possible with regularity to enter and completely inspect the posterolateral compartment; the technique is detailed in Chapter 3. Prior to that, it was thought that an adequate view of that compartment could be achieved from an anterior approach, but direct viewing of the area showed this to be erroneous. Many meniscal lesions in the posterolateral compartment cannot be visualized from the front, even with the small-diameter endoscope. More important, the posterolateral compartment harbors most loose bodies found in the knee joint. Many can be removed through a cannula placed in the compartment. It became apparent that for complete evaluation, posterolateral inspection was required even for patients with normal anterior arthroscopic findings of the lateral compartment.

At this time we were satisfied that it was possible to inspect virtually every recess of the knee joint by direct observation.

DOCUMENTATION
Slide photography

The first photographs made to document arthroscopic observations were taken with a single-reflex camera, using available light from a 300-W source and Kodak high-speed Ektachrome ASA-160 film. The photographs were primitive at best, due to the narrow angle of view of the endoscope, the inability with still photography to create a composition including adjacent areas, and the limited light source. With the improved Model III Needlescope, the problems, except for that of composition, have been resolved.

Because it provides a larger cross-sectional area of fiber light and has a larger diameter lens, the rod-lens scope with attached Storz flash generator produces the best photographic image. Kodachrome 64 film gives the best color balance to the intra-articular tissues.

Cinephotography

Because slides are unsatisfactory for developing composition and because of the low light levels, movie photography provides the best means of documentation. In February 1973, Mr. Harold Neuman matched color film to a light source and provided an optical adaptor from the camera to the endoscope. He had built the original 300-W short-arc lamp illuminator, first known as the Blue Max and now marketed as the Dyonics Model 500 illuminator. The first movies were taken at a rather slow shutter speed with Ektachrome 7241 film. Cinephotography became the medium of choice for documenting technique.

Television

In the spring of 1976, with the utilization of the technology provided by television, it was possible to document more clearly the observations made with the Needlescope. Video equipment could produce an image at a lower light level than was possible with cinephotography. By this time videocassette recordings were being used as a means of transmitting our findings to the referring orthopedists. This allowed them not only a narrative but the same visualization of abnormalities as observed during arthroscopy.

SUMMARY

The comprehensive arthroscopic examination of the knee includes visualization of every recess in the knee joint; posteromedial and posterolateral compartments may be seen, as well as the region beneath the menisci in the area of the coronary ligaments. Further, when there are diagnostic problems this examination is easily performed with patients under local anesthesia. The same technique is adaptable for the complete inspection of the knee joint prior to surgical procedures in those patients for whom clinical diagnosis is established. The technique provides access for synovial membrane biopsy and collection of synovial fluid for microscopic studies. The comprehensive technique includes intra-articular documentation by still and cinephotography or videotape recordings. It has proved to be a simple, efficient, and reliable technique.

REFERENCES

1. Casscells, S. W.: Arthroscopy of the knee joint: a review of 150 cases, J. Bone Joint Surg. (Am.) **53**:287-298, 1971.
2. Eikelaar, H. R.: Arthroscopy of the knee. Groningen, Holland, 1975, Royal United Printers, Hoitsema B. V.
3. Jackson, R. W., and Abe, I.: The role of arthroscopy in the management of disorders of the knee: an analysis of 200 consecutive examinations, J. Bone Joint Surg. (Br.) **54**:310-322, 1972.
4. Jackson, R. W., and DeHaven, K. E.: Arthroscopy of the knee, Clin. Orthop. **107**:87-92, 1975.
5. Johnson, L. L.: Diagnostic arthroscopy of the knee: the knee joint, Amsterdam, Excerpta Medica; New York, 1974, American Elsevier Publishing Co., 131-319.
6. Johnson, L. L.: Arthroscopy of the knee using local anesthesia: a review of 400 patients, J. Bone Joint Surg. (Am.) **58**(5):736, 1976.
7. McGinty, J. B., and Freedman, A.: Arthroscopy of the knee: a review of 221 consecutive cases, J. Bone Joint Surg. (Am.) **54**(5):736, 1976.
8. O'Conner, R.: Arthroscopy in the diagnosis and treatment of acute ligament injuries of the knee, J. Bone Joint Surg. (Am.) **56**:333-337, 1974.
9. Watanabe, M., and Takeda, S.: The number 21 arthroscope, J. Jpn. Orthop. Assoc. **34**:1041, 1960.
10. Watanabe, M.: Arthroscope: present and future, Surg. Ther. **26**(7):73, 1972.

Chapter 2

Instrumentation

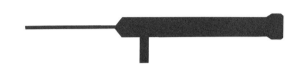

SELECTION OF AN ARTHROSCOPE

The selection of an arthroscope is based on the personality, vision, eye-hand coordination, and technical ability of the arthroscopist. No endoscope is the ideal for every arthroscopist. The initial purchase is usually difficult because limitations of the scope are not recognized. With the second endoscope, a system can be selected that has advantages not possible with the first. All endoscopes or other optical systems have limitations, and trade-offs may be necessary in the purchase of new equipment.

It is possible in selected patients to carry out a complete arthroscopy of the knee with virtually any endoscope, except perhaps the Watanabe No. 21, which is too large with the tungsten light bulb attached. I prefer the 1.7-mm diameter Needlescope, which when housed in its cannula has an outside diameter of 2 mm. This small-diameter endoscope allows ease of access under the menisci and into the posteromedial and posterolateral compartments that the larger diameter endoscopes do not afford. If multiple punctures are made with a large-diameter endoscope (e.g., 3.5-mm), the joint will deflate because of leakage from previous entry sites; when distention is lost, ease of access into the posteromedial and posterolateral compartments is diminished. In some patients, even a 2.2-mm Needlescope with a 2.6-mm cannula limits access for viewing the posterior horn from an anterior approach. With use of large-diameter endoscopes, the view of the knee joint that has normal stability is even more limited, whether the patient is under local or general anesthesia.

TYPES OF ARTHROSCOPES
Thin-lens system

In the classic thin-lens system (Fig. 2-1), the lenses are thin in comparison with their diameters. Air spaces separate each of the conventional lenses. The objective lens is to the left and transmits the light from the image through the relay lens system to the ocular lens. The ocular lens transmits the image to the observer's eye. The Wolfe endoscope is an example of this construction.

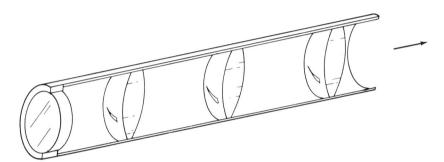

FIG. 2-1. Classic thin-lens system is series of small lenses divided by cylinders of air. Image comes through objective lens from left and is transmitted by relay lens system to ocular lens. Light is transmitted in direction of arrow to arthroscopist's eye. The relay lens system varies in different types of endoscopes.

Rod-lens system

The rod-lens system (Fig. 2-2, *A*) was designed by Professor H. H. Hopkins. In this system the lenses are thick as compared with the diameter. The surfaces are convex, and the air space between the lenses is relatively small. The cylindrical space is glass rather than air, as in the thin-lens relay system. The image is transmitted by the ocular lens to the eyepiece. The Storz-Hopkins rod-lens system (Fig. 2-2, *B*) and Dyonics rod-lens systems (Fig. 2-2, *C* and *D*) are representative.

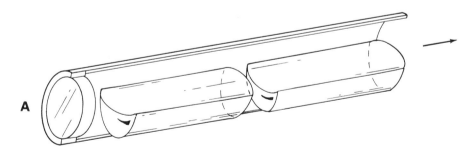

FIG. 2-2. A, Rod-lens system is series of glass cylinders separated by small areas of air, or reverse of thin-lens system. **B,** Storz rod lens system is available in two sizes, with a 2.7-mm telescope or a 4-mm telescope. Both provide excellent optical clarity. **C,** Dyonics rod lens affords excellent optical clarity and has trocar and cannula of simpler design and operation than does Storz endoscope. **D,** *Left to right,* 4.1-mm diameter Dyonics rod lens endoscope; 2.2-mm Needlescope seen in end view; 1.7-mm Needlescope; No. 18 needle, shown for relative size comparison.

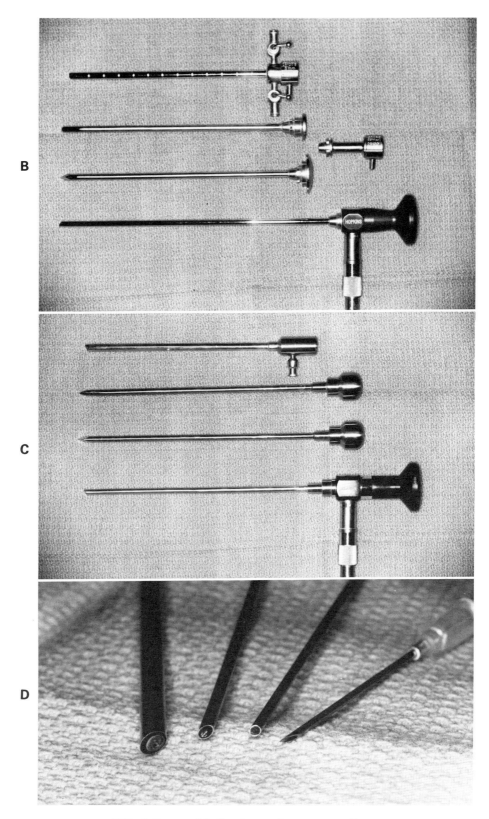

FIG. 2-2, cont'd. For legend see opposite page.

Coherent bundle system

The coherent bundle system (Fig. 2-3) has an objective lens that relays the light from the image. It is then transmitted through a bundle of coherent light fibers. The image is transmitted through the ocular lens to the observer's eye. With this system the viewer sees many fine dots, each of which transmits an element of the image that is being viewed. It is marketed as a No. 24–type arthroscope by the Pro-Med Company.

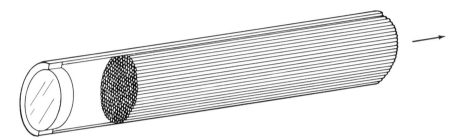

FIG. 2-3. Fused coherent bundle system transmits light by individual fibers. Composition consists of many fine dots, each transmitting an element of image.

Graded refractory index system

A graded refractory index (GRIN) lens system is one in which the entire instrument consists of a slender rod of glass. The refractory index decreases from the center to the periphery according to a specific mathematical relationship. The lens is processed by an ion-exchange treatment utilizing cesium. This endoscope is self-focusing (Selfoc). The rays of light that enter the lens from a particular point in an optic space follow helioid patterns and come into focus, periodically along the rod, producing an image.[1] The Watanabe No. 24 arthroscope (1.7-mm diameter) was the precursor of the Needlescope (Fig. 2-4).

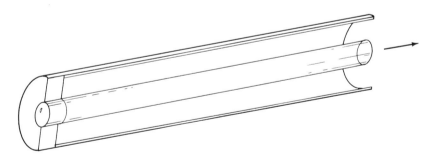

FIG. 2-4. Needlescope system consists of two graded refractory index (GRIN) lenses and an ocular lens. Objective lens, about 3 mm in length and 1 mm in diameter, gives a wide field of view. Relay lens, about 134 mm in length and 1 mm in diameter, transfers image from objective lens back to ocular lens, which magnifies image for viewing.

LIGHT SOURCES

I have utilized a variety of light sources, perhaps virtually every one on the market in North America, in demonstrating the technique of the comprehensive

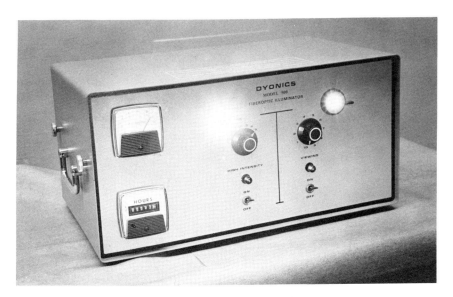

FIG. 2-5. Dyonics Model 500 light source.

arthroscopic examination of the knee. It is my opinion that the Dyonics Model 500 light source (Fig. 2-5) and the Storz xenon arc illuminator are the light sources of choice for the serious arthroscopist. The intensity of the light in these two sources is comparable. The color arc appears different when documented photographically and perhaps would not be apparent to the uninitiated eye. Movie film strips of the same patient taken on the same day, changing only the light source, show the Model 500 illuminator to have a blue-white light, which provides more optical clarity than does the xenon light source, which has a slight yellowish tint. Other light sources that have less intensity can be used, but the depth of field of illumination is limited, as is the clarity, and the photographic capacity is diminished.

LIGHT GUIDES

A variety of light guides, or cables, are available. Any manufacturer will make attachments for a competitor's endoscopes, and vice versa. The Silastic covering on the Dyonics and Wolfe cables is more thermal resistant than is that marketed by others and therefore has a potentially longer life. It has been my experience that cables manufactured by Dyonics last for approximately 1 year and in excess of 300 steam autoclavings. Care of the cables is important; they should not be kinked or twisted. As with any other technical equipment, performance of the light cable should be checked periodically so that gradual deterioration does not compromise the arthroscopic examination. The passage of light or usage over many months does not wear out the cables. However, over a period of time (approximately 1 year) multiple fiber breaks develop, and light cannot be transmitted along the entire length of the cable. To check for breaks, first turn off bright overhead lights; then hold one end of the cable up to an available lamp (light bulb). By looking down the end of the cable, one can visualize darkened or black areas (breaks). Also, that same fiber will emit light at the point of the break along the cable.

ACCESSORIES
Cannulas and forceps

Cannulas may serve various purposes. For the irrigation of joints, a separate cannula is used to provide a source of saline. Section through a second cannula removes multiple loose bodies. For example, if the posterolateral compartment is being viewed and a large number of loose bodies of small diameter are seen in that compartment, a separate cannula, 2 mm in outside diameter, can be placed anteriorly in the joint to deliver fluid to flush them out. Cannulas up to 6.5-mm outside diameter have been utilized for the removal of large loose bodies or for the insertion of a modified pituitary forceps for removal of large loose bodies.

A regular pituitary forceps was originally used for removal of loose bodies; however, the loose body often pinched out of the forceps like a watermelon seed. A reversed-tooth pituitary forceps was designed, called Jaws (Fig. 2-7). Material being removed from a joint should not slip from this instrument. This is especially important with large loose bodies of up to 1 inch in diameter. They can be gripped percutaneously with this instrument. When the forceps holding the loose body is firmly up against the capsule, a local anesthetic can be placed alongside the instrument shaft. An incision is then made, down to the loose body. Stretching of the tissues permits removal of a loose body through an incision smaller than the diameter of the loose body. Ronjeuring of partially attached articular cartilage is also possible during arthroscopic examination. The Jaws forceps may be used during open-knee surgery for grasping small tags of menisci that remain after excision of the major fragment.

A miniature biopsy forceps (Fig. 2-8) can be placed through a 2-mm outside diameter cannula for synovial membrane biopsy. It is possible in cases of diffuse synovitis to excise multiple pieces by this technique without directly visualizing them. A separate puncture will permit biopsy with direct vision.

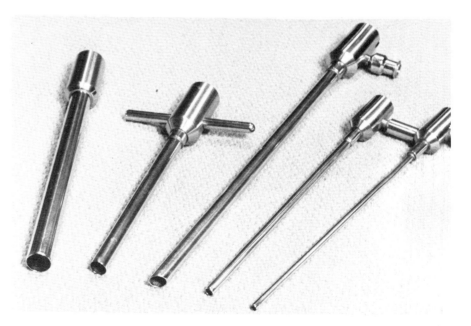

FIG. 2-6. Cannulas varying in size from 8-mm outside diameter *(left)* to 2-mm outside diameter *(right)*. Latter holds a 1.7-mm Needlescope.

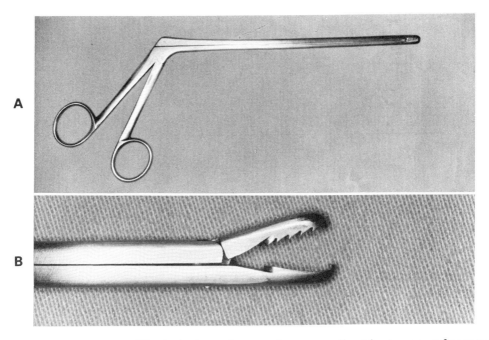

FIG. 2-7. **A,** Jaws modified pituitary forceps is an excellent instrument for removing loose bodies of rather large size, even with patient under local anesthesia. Instrument can be useful in operations where patient requires general anesthetic, for grasping of fragments of menisci that must be excised. **B,** Close-up of reverse-tooth Jaws modified pituitary forceps. Notice reversed teeth superiorly, which guard against slippage of loose body. Scooped-out inferior portion of forceps is for holding oval-shaped foreign body.

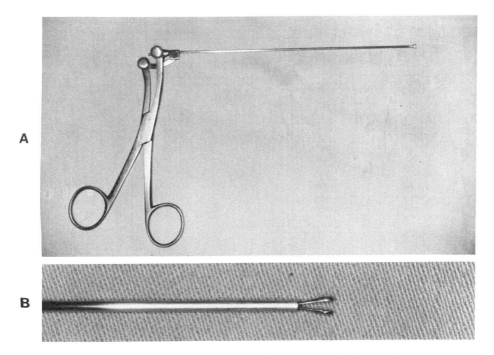

FIG. 2-8. **A,** Small biopsy forceps can be placed through 2-mm diameter cannula of Needlescope. Biopsy can be done by a separate puncture under direct vision or blindly through existing puncture. **B,** Biting end of miniature biopsy forceps.

Halo light

Fragility of the small-diameter endoscope (1.7-mm outside diameter) has been of concern, especially in training programs. Therefore, the halo light, or teaching cannula, was introduced (Fig. 2-9). This 3.5-mm outside diameter cannula provides 16 times the illumination of the small-diameter Needlescope. It allows arthroscopists to become proficient with the small-diameter scope and yet have the safety, protection, and photographic capacity of a larger diameter endoscope.

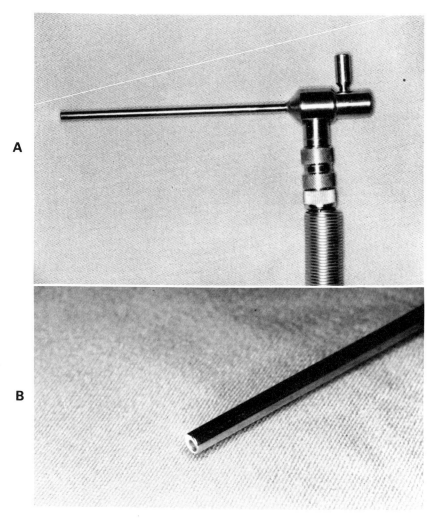

FIG. 2-9. A, Halo light is advantageous for photographic work and for protection of small-diameter endoscope when utilized for training purposes. **B,** End of halo light. Notice central opening that will house 1.7-mm Needlescope. Illumination is up to 16 times that of endoscope.

Light wand

A light wand (Fig. 2-10) is helpful in transillumination and photographic work. It is placed either parallel to the view or may transilluminate tissue for examination. Transillumination first showed the engulfing of saline by synovium. Observation of the vascular pattern and morphologic characteristics is enhanced by transillumination effects on photographic film.

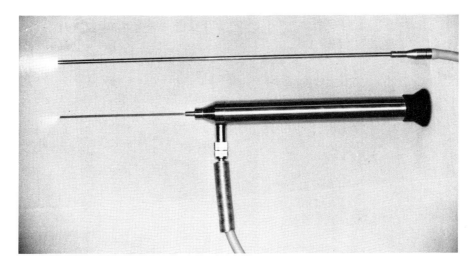

FIG. 2-10. Light wand, shown above Needlescope, can be useful for photographic purposes, especially transillumination. It is brought into knee through a separate puncture wound. Photographs are taken through small-diameter endoscope with a camera attached to ocular lens.

STERILIZATION AND DISINFECTION

Sterilization of endoscopic equipment has caused considerable concern among orthopedic surgeons and nursing personnel. Sterile technique and the prevention of infection are essential.

No arthroscope will withstand high-pressure steam autoclaving indefinitely. The present construction of arthroscopes is such that with this type of sterilization the adhesive seals between the lenses or the chambers eventually breaks down. Therefore, it is recommended that the endoscope be sterilized with ethyline oxide gas. One of the disadvantages of this method of sterilization is that many hospitals do not possess the necessary equipment. In addition, it takes at least 4 hours, sometimes overnight, for complete drying after the sterilization process. This is very impractical because the arthroscopist is restricted to one examination per arthroscope per day. One is not likely to purchase a number of expensive instruments in order that more than one arthroscopic procedure can be carried out each day. Therefore, an alternate method of sterilization that is practical and safe must be found.

Our method of disinfection is to first clean the endoscope with alcohol and then place it in activated dialdehyde solution (Cidex) for 20 minutes. Prior to use, it is rinsed with sterile saline; when dry, it is placed on a sterile Mayo stand. Other equipment used for arthroscopy (i.e., cannulas, light cords, catheters, and suction tubes) are either steam autoclavable or are disposable sterile materials.

At the close of each week, all the equipment is cleaned, assembled for ethyline oxide sterilization over the weekend, and stored.

In my experience over the past 4 years with nearly 2,000 patients, no infection or hepatitis has resulted. For one 18-month period in which over 400 patients were arthroscopically examined, either under local or general anesthesia, ethyline oxide sterilization was not utilized, but the endoscopes were cleansed with Cidex disinfectant only. No patients developed infection. Some patients experienced "unexplained" synovitis either after surgery or arthroscopy. Cultures were taken, but none showed positive findings. Most cases of synovitis were nonspecific, with negative culture findings. Some occurred secondary to articular loose bodies within the joint; cleansing the joint of the loose bodies or synovial debris remedied the synovitis.

Most arthroscopists use a disinfection method similar to that described above in order to facilitate doing a series of arthroscopies in one day. There has been no attempt, to my knowledge, to incur the rigors of an Environmental Protection Agency investigation to validate the use of activated dialdehyde solution (Cidex) for cold sterilization in arthroscopy. When this chemical was introduced in 1964, the label indicated that a 3-hour sterilization time was appropriate. This was based on the spore-testing method accepted by the United States Department of Agriculture, which regulated such things as pesticides and disinfectants, and which at the time used stainless steel penicylinders. In 1969 the responsibility for evaluation of pesticides and disinfectants was transferred to the Environmental Protection Agency. That agency employs a loop-suture method for spore testing, which requires that a sterilization solution penetrate the fibers of the loop material as well as the spore itself. Because loop fibers are more difficult to penetrate than is stainless steel, the required sterilization time for Cidex became 10 hours, indicated on the chemical's label. There has been no provision made by the Environmental Protection Agency for a method that would be comparable to soaking arthroscopes or laparoscopes in Cidex for between 10 and 30 minutes. However, no instance of infection as a result of this technique has been reported to the manufacturer. The bulk of clinical evidence supports Cidex disinfecting as safe and practical, and it is the standard of practice of established arthroscopists throughout the United States.

REFERENCES

1. Prescott, R.: Optical principles of endoscopy, J. Med. Primatol. **5**(2):133-147, 1976.
2. Arbrook Inc., Arlington, Texas: personal correspondence, 1976.

Technique

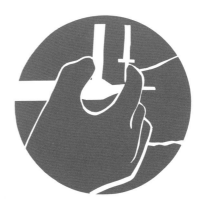

The comprehensive arthroscopic examination of the knee requires that established principles and disciplines be used to successfully accomplish the technique.

Although arthroscopy is potentially a simple procedure, a great number of details need attention before the technique is accomplished with ease. As orthopedists, we are accustomed to working with tools. In recent years new operative procedures (i.e., Harrington rod instrumentation or total-hip surgery) have required increased focus of attention on a number of details heretofore not required in the usual orthopedic surgical procedures. Although arthroscopy does not require that an incision be made or that anatomic pathways be known, there is no decrease in the technical details to be attended to nor any less demand on the technical prowess of the surgeon. The procedure demands mastering the use of a fine instrument, the arthroscope.

Preoperative organization and planning will contribute more to the technical skill with which the procedure is accomplished than will any compensatory effort during arthroscopy. It is important that procedures be done in a similar manner each time. Each member of the arthroscopic team performs his or her duties in coordination with the others in a similar manner for every operation. Responsibilities do not overlap, and there is very little improvisation. Each participant has a great deal of individual responsibility, carried out with the support of the other members of the team. Such compulsiveness may bother some personalities, but it eliminates aimlessness during the surgical procedure.

TECHNICAL CONCEPTS

A number of concepts are unique to arthroscopy and must be mastered by any physician desiring to become an accomplished arthroscopist. I have learned many of the technical details by trial and error. The following narrative is offered so that others may learn more easily.

Placement

Excellent placement of the endoscope is essential to successful arthroscopy. A scope placed too superiorly does not enter the slot of the intercondylar space, and access for viewing the posterior horn is eliminated. It is possible that a scope placed too inferiorly could go through or under the meniscus, impeding movement and limiting subsequent viewing (Fig. 3-1). Uninitiated arthroscopists are so intense about initial placement that they fail to see that an incorrect positioning should be redone. It is considered good technique to redirect or replace rather than to waste time twisting and wrestling with a badly positioned arthroscope.

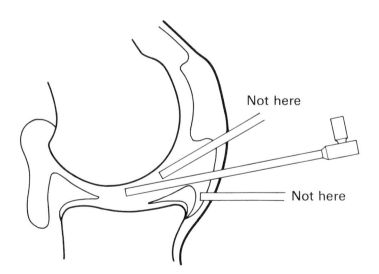

FIG. 3-1. Ideal placement of cannula. If positioned too high, angle of obliquity is such that posterior horn cannot be seen; if too low, it can go through meniscus and limit visualization or mobility. Ideal placement is directly in slot between femur and tibia.

18

Entrée

It is advantageous that the endoscope enter the suprapatellar pouch rather briskly and then be retracted very slowly. Brisk entry allows the synovium to hang up on the shank of the metallic cannula, and slow retraction of the instrument prevents the fat pad from slipping down over the end of the scope, which makes intra-articular viewing impossible (Fig. 3-2).

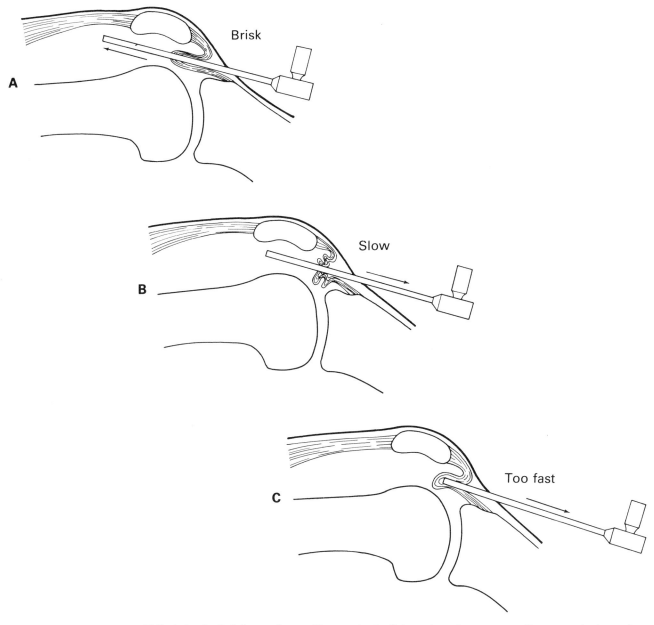

FIG. 3-2. A, Brisk motion will penetrate fat pad and suprapatellar pouch, hanging fat pad synovium on shank of cannula. **B,** Very slow retraction of cannula and endoscope will prevent fat pad from slipping over end of scope. **C,** Fast retraction will pull endoscope into fat pad and obscure viewing.

For the uninitiated arthroscopist, it is important that the inside of the joint be visualized before any fluid is instilled, to be certain that entry has been accomplished. Fluid placed outside the capsule only compresses the potential space of the knee joint and impedes subsequent viewing.

After entry has been confirmed, the joint is distended (Fig. 3-3), or it may be distended with a separate needle prior to entry. If the joint is not filled with any obscuring synovial fluid or blood, viewing may commence. At this time the operating room lights are turned out; the x-ray viewbox provides sufficient illumination for activity in the room but does not distract the arthroscopist.

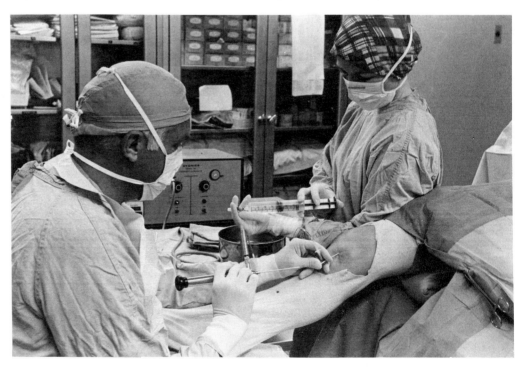

FIG. 3-3. After penetration has been confirmed, trocar is removed from cannula. Arthroscopist places thumb over end of cannula, and assistant forces approximately 60 ml of normal saline through polyethylene catheter into joint. With this maximal distention, viewing can commence.

Replacement

It is not necessary to make another stab wound through the skin. Replacement can be accomplished by pulling the cannula and trocar out through the capsule, then elevating them 1 or 2 mm or moving them from side to side 1 or 2 mm, thus gaining access to the intercondylar slot (Fig. 3-4).

Redirection

It is important that the initial entry be at a 30° angle toward the lateral side (Fig. 3-4). In a knee that is fat (with a large fulcrum) or scarred (with a rigid fulcrum), redirection may be necessary. In unusual circumstances, such as in a tight, fat, or scarred joint, it may be necessary to redirect as many as three times in order to view one compartment. In most cases, after viewing in the suprapatellar pouch, lateral compartment, and intercondylar notch through the original placement, the medial compartment can be entered, but bending of the scope may occur. Redirection to the area of the medial meniscus attachment is simple, painless, and nondestructive and facilitates completion of the examination of the anterior and superior chambers.

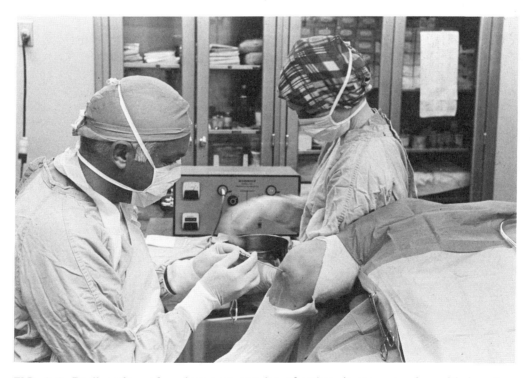

FIG. 3-4. Redirection of endoscope can be of value. It may require withdrawing, reinserting cannula, and moving as little as 1 mm superiorly or laterally in order to achieve exact position. It is considered good technique to redirect endoscope. This is most often necessary when viewing in medial compartment in a patient who has a scarred or fat knee with a large fulcrum.

Hand control

The endoscope is held very firmly with the index finger and thumb (Fig. 3-5), although the wrist and upper arm should be relaxed to facilitate movement of the scope. The firmness of grip allows precise movements and prevents slippage. Dexterity is provided by the combined universal joints of the wrist, elbow, and shoulder. Lack of precision in holding an endoscope, cannula, or trocar will result in quick motions and potential abrasions to the knee joint or injury to the endoscope.

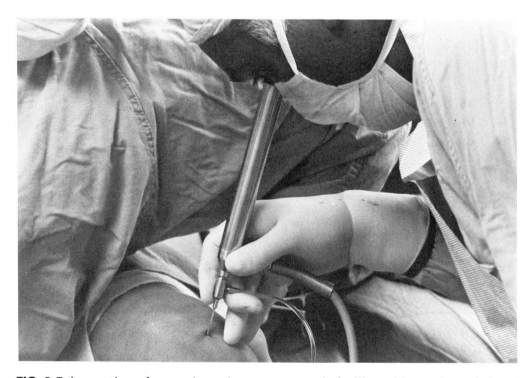

FIG. 3-5. Inspection of anterolateral compartment is facilitated by assistant's hand held to the medial distal femur and valgus force being applied by arthroscopist. Notice safe distance between arthroscopist's hand and viewing eyepiece; this reduces contamination. Endoscope is securely held. Middle finger holds cannula tight against arthroscope, which facilitates manipulation without loosening grip.

Palpation

Although arthroscopy emphasizes hand-eye coordination, palpation skill is important. As technical skills improve, so does ability to sense by palpation a location within the knee joint. Visualization follows. For instance, one learns to sense by drag and palpation the different layers of fat, capsule, and synovium, that have been penetrated, as well as the position of the endoscope in relation to the patella and the suprapatellar pouch. After some experience, the anterior cruciate ligament can be sensed without direct visualization.

A well-placed scope and an awareness of palpation will result in an excellent arthroscopic examination.

REMEMBER: PLACEMENT, PALPATION, THEN VISUALIZATION

Manipulation

Manipulation of the scope in the knee joint is best facilitated with the assistant stabilizing the knee, either with her elbow on the lateral side or her hand on the inner side (Fig. 3-2). Some patients tend to roll, externally rotating the hip; thus stabilization of the thigh is essential to placement and manipulation of the endoscope. With experience, the assistant and the arthroscopist will learn to coordinate their efforts so that a good position is accomplished for endoscope viewing and documentation on film.

Distention

Distention of the joint is essential and may be accomplished by filling the knee through a separate needle puncture or after direct entry with the endoscope by the more experienced arthroscopist. Entry should be confirmed by direct visualization prior to the instillation of saline. Whichever method is used for joint distention, extravasation of fluid outside of the joint should not be allowed, because it will compress the potential space of the joint. The synovium will absorb approximately 25 ml of saline every 5 minutes. Therefore, the distended joint will collapse after a short period of viewing. Instillation of another bolus of 50 ml of saline is required for maximal retraction of the synovium and capsule wall. With close arthroscopic inspection the saline can be seen engulfed in the synovial villae, appearing very much like silver or translucent balls (the saline) within larger balloons (the synovial villae). This commences quite quickly after instillation of the saline and continues throughout the procedure. Prolonged use of separate drainage tubes for instillation of saline under pressure results in considerable absorption of fluid, increased thickness of the synovium, and capsular edema. There is some decreased mobility and increased morbidity following this method of irrigation.

Distention is paramount in making the posteromedial and posterolateral entries for the comprehensive examination of the joint. The use of the small-diameter endoscope reduces the leakage about the previous puncture sites, and there is less loss of distention.

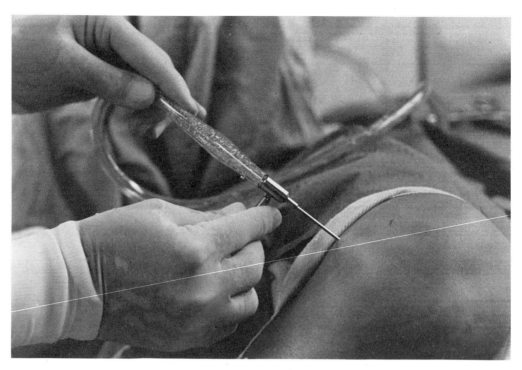

FIG. 3-6. Vacuuming of joint to cleanse it of loose bodies and bloody synovial debris is often indicated. Notice that plastic tubing is slightly open and angulated at cannula entrance so as not to create a complete vacuum, bringing synovium up to tip of cannula inside joint. With slight break in suction, it is possible to cleanse joint very well for perfect viewing.

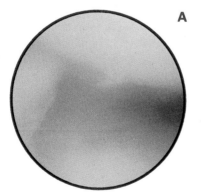
A

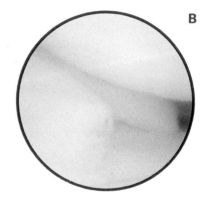
B

FIG. 3-7. A, Arthroscopic photograph taken prior to cleansing of cloudy synovial fluid in joint. **B,** After vacuuming synovial debris from joint and reinstilling clear bolus of saline, arthroscopic visualization is much clearer.

Cleansing and vacuuming

It should be emphasized that the best photographic results are obtained in a clean joint. Cleansing is accomplished by directly vacuuming out any synovial fluid, debris, or blood that may be in the joint (Fig. 3-6). Jackson reported that hemarthrosis was a contraindication to arthroscopy. With drainage tubes and recirculation of fluid, blood in the joint can be gradually diluted, but not enough that visualization is quickly and readily accomplished. The joint with hemarthrosis can be completely cleansed of blood-tinged synovial fluid by vacuuming through the cannula (Fig. 3-7). As the endoscope is moved from one compartment to another, blood may run from one recess of the joint to another and cloud the compartment. Repeat vacuuming with the cannula may be necessary in each compartment to be examined. A bolus of saline will sweep material out of the way for excellent viewing.

It may be necessary to clean proteinaceous material off the end of the scope or to clear an area of syrupy synovial fluid that is interfering with viewing. This can be accomplished by instilling saline through a K-52 catheter placed adjacent to the endoscope.

Vacuuming of a joint can be therapeutic in that pieces of articular cartilage and synovial debris are removed (Fig. 3-7). The force of the suction will remove pieces of softened articular cartilage larger than the diameter of the endoscope, because they fold on themselves and are drawn out through the cannula. Larger, firmer pieces that contain bone must be removed by a Jaws modified pituitary forceps (see Fig. 11-2, *C*).

Contrast staining

The use of contrast dye during arthroscopy was reported by Burman[1] and reviewed recently by Guten.[2] Methylene blue has not produced any complications in over 100 of my patients. It readily clears from the joint and has no permanent sequelae. It can be of benefit in arthroscopy because it demonstrates morphologic characteristics of the articular surfaces or synovium. It has been of special benefit in diagnosing osteochondritis dissecans (see Fig. 11-2, *A* and *B*) and in the study of synovial diseases (see Fig. 13-1, *C* to *E*). Staining has been most valuable in those patients with diffuse degenerative arthritis, which has a shaggy, wooly arthroscopic appearance. Optically ill-defined borders diminish definition of the contours of the articular cartilage and meniscus. Methylene blue increases contrast in joints with these degenerative changes and enhances diagnostic capabilities.

Scanning the horizon

As in surgery, it is important to work from known to unknown. Where there is no known identifiable structure, the arthroscopist must return to the area that was last identified and then progress to areas yet to be documented. One of the most important landmarks arthroscopically is the tangential horizon of the femoral condyle. It is possible to move from the patellar surface to the lateral femoral condyle and follow it tangentially all the way to the lateral compartment. As the horizon is followed, the edge of the meniscus will come into view. It is then possible by repositioning of the knee and the scope to follow the inner margin of the meniscus all the way to the posterior horn.

Pistoning

The back and forth motion of the endoscope can be described as pistoning. Pistoning can establish location and dimension, and the size of the object being viewed can be conceptualized in relation to other objects (see Fig. 6-5).

Rotation

I prefer, as do many arthroscopists, an endoscope with a fore-oblique view, that is, approximately 30° off center (Fig. 3-8). With such a scope it is possible to view directly as well as slightly to the side. This is essential in the knee joint, where after placement of the scope most objects are to the side (i.e., the meniscus) or above or below (i.e., the patella and intercondylar notch). It is not difficult with a minimum of practice with a fore-oblique viewing device to become accustomed to this angle of viewing. The other advantage of a fore-oblique viewing device is that with rotation one may view in an opposite direction than that being observed. Without change in position, the scope can be rotated, moving the image to the right or to the left. Rotation of the fore-oblique scope, therefore, increases the range of viewing, which is not accomplished as satisfactorily with rotation of a direct-viewing scope with the same optical angle of view.

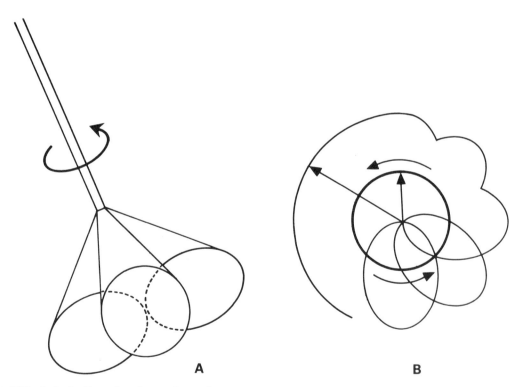

FIG. 3-8. A, Result of rotation of direct-viewing device in center, which is essentially a circle. When circle is rotated, view does not change. When fore-oblique endoscope is rotated, view changes from one side to the opposite side, and effective viewing area is increased. **B,** Comparison of end-on view of diameter of straight-viewing endoscope versus fore-oblique endoscope. Notice considerable increase in area and diameter of view possible with fore-oblique scope when rotated.

Scope sweeping

Another basic manipulative principle involves motion of the scope (Fig. 3-9). If a stick 4 inches long has a fulcrum in the middle, there are 2 inches on each side of it. If one end of the stick is displaced 1 inch, the opposite end is also displaced 1 inch. Likewise, when an endoscope is displaced rather rapidly at one end (outside the knee) a rather broad arc is made at the opposite end (inside). The ratio, of course, is not equal, because length outside the knee is greater than inside. Gross movements of the scope during repositioning or viewing should be guarded against because the tip of the endoscope may be displaced from ½ to 1 inch within the joint.

When a scope is moved very slowly a natural sequence of images is observed. Although there is no depth perception because the scope has a single ocular lens, slow movements, combined with the above-described manipulative procedures, make it possible to fully comprehend the arthroscopic composite.

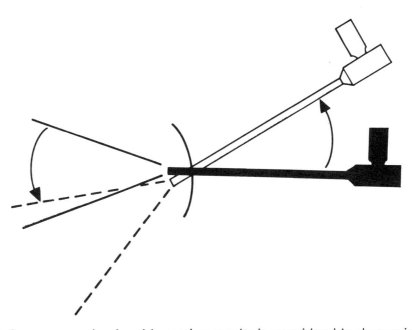

FIG. 3-9. Scope sweeping in wide motion results in considerable change in objective viewed. It is important to realize that rather gross outside motion with endoscope produces marked change in angle of view inside knee; therefore, rather gentle scanning motions slowly performed are indicated for best viewing.

Free hand activity

The arthroscopist holds the endoscope in one hand and the patient's ankle in the other (Fig. 3-10). With patients under local anesthesia it is possible to monitor the tightness of the lower extremity by their spontaneous tightening of the Achilles tendon. Varus and valgus strain or rotational stress can be applied to the joint in coordination with positioning of the endoscope to create a good arthroscopic image. One hand can be freed for scope manipulation, vacuuming, or suctioning by resting the patient's leg against the hip, while the assistant supplies support. For lateral viewing or vacuuming, the arthroscopist can use his free hand to bring the patient's foot into his lap and with support being provided to the inner side by the assistant, push the patient's knee into the varus position.

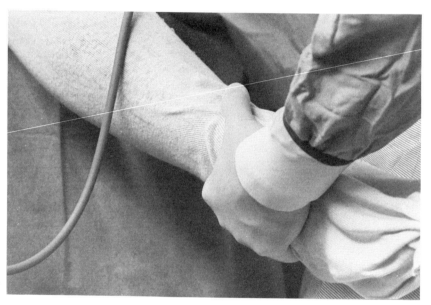

FIG. 3-10. With free hand, arthroscopist can hold patient's ankle and monitor tightening of Achilles tendon. Any tightening of knee or apprehension of patient is very quickly discerned by Achilles tendon tenseness, allowing arthroscopist to be sensitive to the patient's comfort under local anesthesia. In addition, with internal and external rotation, flexion and extension, abduction and adduction, arthroscopist can compose clear-cut endoscopic picture.

TEAM APPROACH

It is important that each member of the arthroscopic team understands his or her delegated responsibilities and participates in a cooperative manner. For example, efforts of the surgeon (e.g., placement of hands for manipulation of the patient's knee) and of the assistant (e.g., positioning of body for support) should be coordinated in a similar manner for each arthroscopy. These habit patterns need not be rigidly observed, but do result in extreme efficiency. Our organizational setup is demonstrated in Fig. 3-11.

All personnel must be familiar with each piece of equipment to be utilized (see box below), and for all procedures these implements should be placed in the same location on the appropriate table.

If each procedure is carried out in a consistent manner, the end results will be more satisfying, with predictable success.

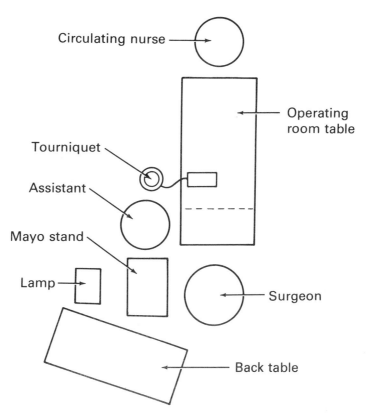

FIG. 3-11. Equipment distribution.

Mayo stand	Back table
1 Straight Mayo scissors	5 Drawsheets
1 No. 11 blade	1 Suction tube
1 No. 3 knife handle	Sponges, 3- × 4-inch
1 Cannula	5 Folded towels
1 Trocar	1 Mayo cover
1 Obturator	1 Polyethylene shield
1 K-52 catheter (Novex three-way	1 Stockinette, 6-inch
stopcock with extension tube)	1 Kling, 4-inch
1 Syringe, 60-ml	1 Preparation tray
1 Small metal basin	6 Towel clips
1 No. 21 needle, 1½-inch	1 Sponge stick
1 Syringe, 12-ml	Lidocaine, 1% plain
1 Light cord	**Head of table**
1 Arthroscope	1 Specimen trap
	1 Pneumatic tourniquet

Circulating nurse

The responsibilities of the circulating nurse are outlined below. Foremost is monitoring of the patient's comfort and vital signs. Conversation with the patient under local anesthesia can contribute to patient assurance and relaxation.

RESPONSIBILITIES OF CIRCULATING NURSE

During set up
1. Turn on lights
2. Set up skin preparation materials
3. Position suction tubing and collection jars for cell-block preparation
4. Open main pack
5. Bring patient into room and position on table so that knees are at edge of table
6. Check and record patient's pulse, blood pressure, and respiration rate
7. Check tourniquet and apply to appropriate thigh
8. Bring in autoclaved instruments; place on opened back table
9. Hold patient's leg during skin preparation
10. Inflate tourniquet
11. Attach light source

During arthroscopy
1. Record patient's blood pressure
2. Converse with patient
3. Collect cell-block specimen and reestablish suction
4. Control light sources

After procedure
1. Deflate tourniquet
2. Record patient's vital signs
3. Label specimen and records
4. Take patient to recovery room
5. Help clean room and set up for next examination

Assistant

The duties of the assistant are outlined below. Among other advantages, coordinated efforts of the surgeon and the assistant facilitate opening of the compartments of the knee. The assistant can cleanse the joint during the procedure, allowing the physician to concentrate on viewing. She stabilizes the patient's thigh, freeing the surgeon's hands and aiding in the patient's comfort and relaxation. By having the assistant assemble and care for equipment, the arthroscopist is able to interact with the patient or document the procedure between cases, increasing efficiency and productivity. As a result of these efforts, we are able to do an arthroscopy, including room change and instrument preparation time, in ½ hour.

RESPONSIBILITIES OF ASSISTANT

During setup
1. Set up back table
2. Set up Mayo stand
3. Assist in preparing and draping patient

During arthroscopy
1. Stabilize patient's knee
2. Handle instruments or pass them to surgeon
3. Keep syringe filled with saline for delivery on command
4. Hand dressings to physician

After procedure
1. Clean equipment
2. Ready steam autoclaving tray
3. Sterilize scope in Cidex
4. Remove and strip operating room of laundry and waste and prepare for next patient

At end of day
1. Clean, dry, and place scope in properly secured compartment

At end of week
1. Prepare arthroscope for gas sterilization

Care of instruments between patients

After each arthroscopic examination, the assistant carefully cleanses the arthroscope with alcohol and places it in activated dialdehyde solution (Cidex). The interior of the cannula is cleaned by forcing saline through it with a K-52 catheter. Other instruments, including all metal tools and the light cable and connectors, are cleaned with saline and alcohol, placed in the sterilization tray, and autoclaved.

Care of endoscopic equipment is important to its longevity. With careful handling, a Needlescope has lasted for 3 years and approximately 300 examinations.

Procedure

A sequential approach to the arthroscopic examination is important.

The circulating nurse inflates the tourniquet. The patient's skin is prepared and the extremity draped (Fig. 3-12). A folded towel is placed under the distal thigh to suspend the knee above the table and facilitate movement (Fig. 3-13). The foot of the operating room table is lowered so that the patient's legs hang down, with knees flexed. She then moves the illuminator into place and attaches the cord to the light source.

The surgeon takes his place at the end of the table and rests the patient's foot in his lap, which is covered with a sterile apron. The Mayo stand is positioned next to him (Fig. 3-14).

The assistant takes a position adjacent to the knee to be examined and helps stabilize the patient's thigh. During the procedure she hands instruments to the surgeon and maintains organization and placement of the instruments on the back table and Mayo stand, enabling the arthroscopist to find equipment in the dim light.

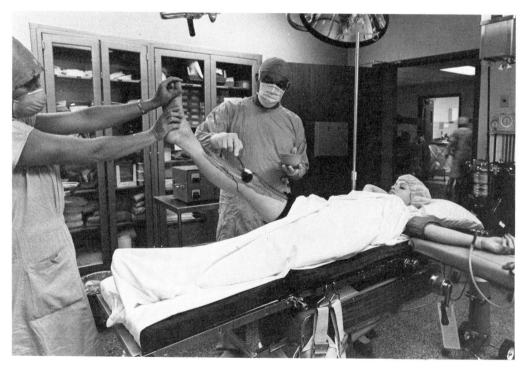

FIG. 3-12. Under local anesthesia, patient is relaxed. Simple skin preparation of povidone-iodine complex (Betadine) is used. Notice that tourniquet is in place but not elevated at this time. With general anesthetic, more elaborate skin preparation and draping is indicated.

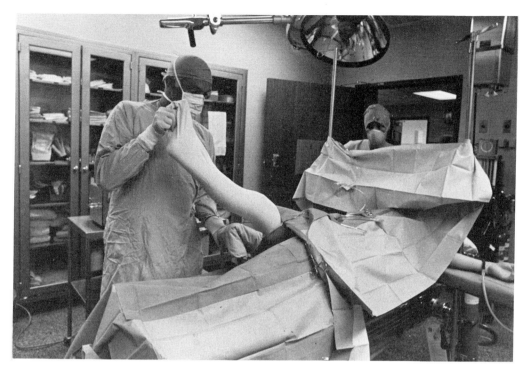

FIG. 3-13. After simple paper drape has been placed on patient's leg, folded towel is placed under knee to provide suspension of knee and greater mobility for arthroscopic inspection.

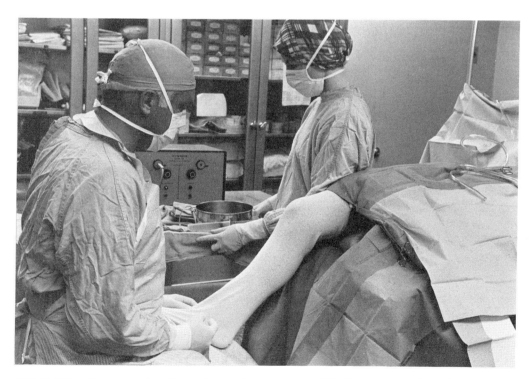

FIG. 3-14. Arthroscopist sits at foot of operating table. Patient is relaxed, with knee hanging freely over end of table. Knee, which would tend to roll into external rotation, is secured by assistant's elbow and weight of her body.

ARTHROSCOPIC COMPARTMENTS

I generally make an anteromedial puncture and view the patellar surface and suprapatellar pouch from below, then move in sequence to the anterolateral compartment, the intercondylar notch, and the anteromedial compartment. At the completion of the anterior viewing, a suprapatellar puncture may be required to observe this area in patients who have a large fulcrum due to fat or a tight scarred capsule or osteophytes around the patella.

Even in patients with normal anteromedial or anterolateral compartments, as viewed in the above sequence, the posterior compartments are inspected, because of their high yield of lesions and loose bodies not seen anteriorly (see Chapter 5).

The posterior approach is not necessary when an abnormality that requires surgical repair is seen in the anterior compartment, because the surgical technique includes an incision that allows routine inspection of the posterior compartment.

Anteromedial approach

An anteromedial entry allows the arthroscopist to sit squarely in front of the patient's extremity. The site is more central in relationship to the knee joint than is a lateral entry, and access to the lateral compartment from the medial side is easier than is viewing posteromedially from an anterior entry. The anteroposterior diameter of the medial condyle is greater than is that of the lateral condyle. Also, with a varus strain on the knee and an anteromedial placement of the endoscope, the knee rotates in such a way that the posterolateral portion of the knee comes forward. Viewing is much easier than in the posteromedial compartment, which is tighter and in a normal stable knee has less opening and anterior rotation. Also, the anteromedial approach is more easily blocked with local anesthetic by infiltration of the infrapatellar branch of the saphenous nerve (Fig. 3-15).

With the patient's knee in a position of 90° flexion and resting in the surgeon's lap (Fig. 3-16), a site of entry is selected one finger breadth above the tibial spine and one-half finger breadth medial to the patellar tendon. This is accomplished by the placement of the index finger against the patellar tendon and down onto the tibial condyle (Fig. 3-17). The skin immediately above the palpating index finger is lanced with a No. 11 blade, and the subcutaneous tissue and capsule are penetrated by a cannula with a sharp trocar. The plane is parallel to the tibial condyles and directed 30° toward the lateral side of the joint. The sharp trocar is exchanged for a blunt one, and the patient's knee is brought into extension. The blunt trocar in the cannula can penetrate the suprapatellar pouch by angling laterally and superiorly (Fig. 3-18). It may be difficult to gain access to the suprapatellar space with this maneuver in some patients who have a scar from previous surgery or a fat knee, because the fulcrum may be limited by the firmness of the scar or the depth of the fat, or in patients with marked osteochondritic prominences about the patella. A separate suprapatellar puncture is indicated in such patients.

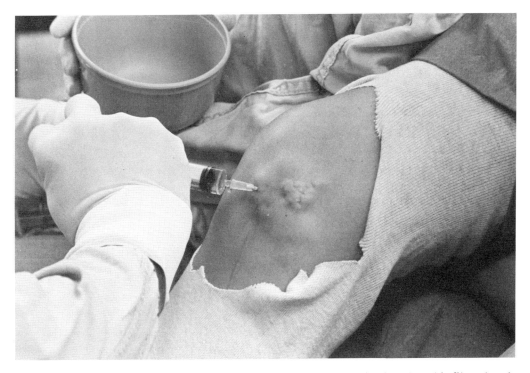

FIG. 3-15. Infrapatellar branch of saphenous nerve is blocked by local infiltration in three to four directions medial from the initial puncture. This decreases proprioception patient might sense during manipulation of knee and therefore reduces apprehension.

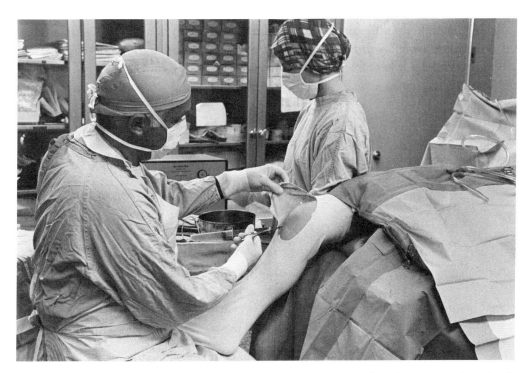

FIG. 3-16. For surgery with local anesthetic, paper barrier drapes and a single stockinette are utilized. If surgical procedure is anticipated, richer draping system is used.

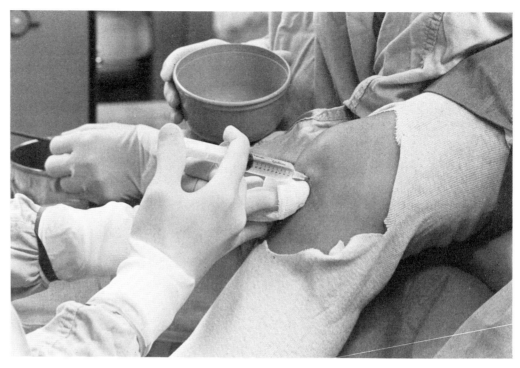

FIG. 3-17. Plain lidocaine, 1%, is placed within knee along course of anticipated penetration of joint. Surgeon places index finger against patellar tendon and onto tibial plateau to palpate for entry one finger breadth above tibial plateau and approximately half a finger breadth medial to inner border of patellar tendon. In some overweight patients, position may be considerably more lateral, because knee tends to rotate externally.

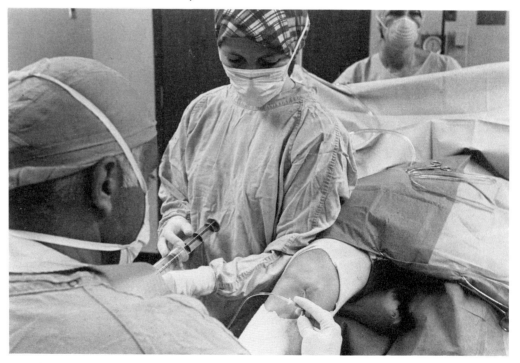

FIG. 3-18. With a blunt trocar in cannula and knee in extension, penetration of suprapatellar pouch is possible. In relaxed patient, patella will float, facilitating entry. Notice that cannula is aligned at an angle of about 30° off center.

Patella and suprapatellar pouch

The assistant stabilizes the lateral femur with her elbow. The physician extends the patient's leg and moves the cannula and blunt trocar into the suprapatellar pouch under the patella. When the patient is relaxed under local anesthesia, flexion and extension allow the patella to float, facilitating entry to this area.

Viewing is then carried out by slowly retracting the endoscope while the leg is extended (Fig. 3-19). By rotating the scope so the inclined view is superior, the horizon of the patella will come into view. From that position, it is possible to scan the patellar surface. The assistant may manipulate the patella so as to bring it into various views for inspection. The suprapatellar pouch can be viewed by advancement of the endoscope. Close inspection of the villae is possible. Plicae, loose bodies, or fibrous adhesions can also be observed. In some patients, the endoscope can be retracted enough that the intercondylar notch and patella can be viewed.

The move to the anterolateral compartment can be facilitated by (1) observing the lateral femoral condyle in tangential view down into the compartment; (2) removing the endoscope, replacing the blunt trocar, and carrying the cannula with the trocar down into the lateral compartment by palpation (this may be especially helpful to the inexperienced arthroscopist who is concerned about fragility of the endoscope during manipulation); or (3) bringing the endoscope tip down into the intercondylar notch and then finding the lateral femoral condyle adjacent to the anterior cruciate ligament. In some patients, there is a large inperforate fat pad up to the ligamentous mucosa. Either direct penetration through this fibrous membrane or moving above the ligamentum mucosum and down into the lateral compartment is required.

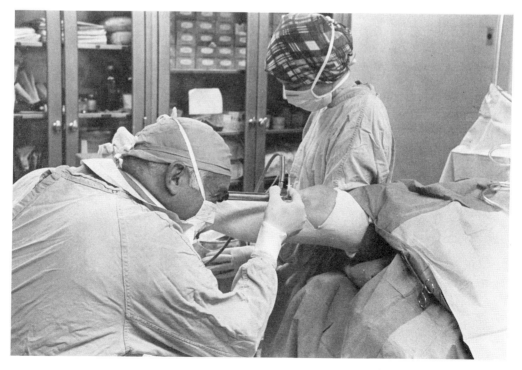

FIG. 3-19. After entry has been confirmed and saline has distended joint, suprapatellar pouch and patellar area may be visualized.

Anterolateral compartment

The anterolateral compartment is best viewed with the patient's knee flexed between 5° and 15°, while the assistant provides support to the medial aspect of the distal femur and the surgeon applies varus strain with his hand on the patient's ankle (Fig. 3-20). If this is accompanied by slight internal rotation of the tibia, the lateral compartment will come into view and the entire meniscus can be visualized easily (see Fig. 7-2, A). It is possible to pass under the posterolateral corner of the meniscus and view the popliteus tendon as it crosses through the open space in the coronary ligament. This tendon appears cordlike and shows a different color reflection than does the meniscus or the tibial condyle (see Fig. 7-2, B). It is important to inspect the lateral reflection of the meniscus at its synovial junction and to follow the tangential view of the condyle at least one meniscus breadth superior to the meniscal-synovial junction. A lesion in this area is pathognomonic of a subluxed or dislocated patella (see Fig. 10-1, B).

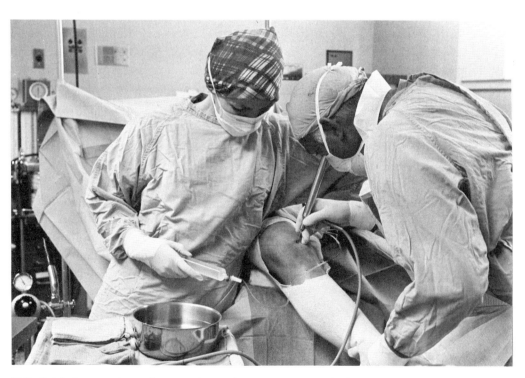

FIG. 3-20. Inspection of anterolateral compartment is facilitated by assistant supporting distal medial femur. Arthroscopist provides varus stress with hand on patient's ankle. Notice that assistant has syringe of saline ready to clear any proteinaceous material from end of scope.

Intercondylar notch

The intercondylar notch is viewed next, with the patient's knee flexed between 45° and 90° and with the assistant stabilizing the lateral femur with her elbow (Fig. 3-21). In this position the anterior cruciate ligament will be in the midportion of the field. In a well-distended knee, the fat pad should not present any problem to entry from the medial side. If the fat pad slips down over the shank of the cannula, a rather smooth but brisk forward motion followed by slow retraction will again hang the fat pad up on the shank of the cannula (Fig. 3-1). Movement across the intercondylar notch is from the femoral condyle on one side around the cruciate ligament to the femoral condyle on the opposite side (see Fig. 7-2, A to C).

It should be noted that at about this point in the procedure there may be some deflation of the distended joint, and instillation of another bolus of saline may be necessary.

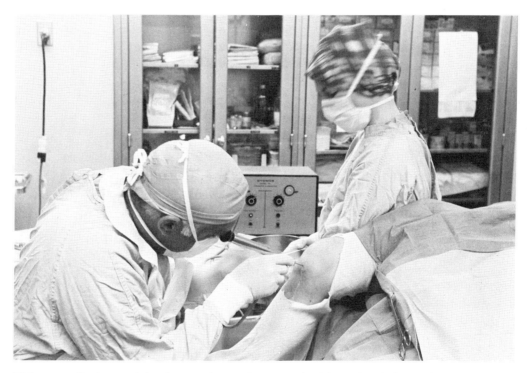

FIG. 3-21. Endocondylar inspection is facilitated with patient's knee flexed approximately 45° to 90°. Arthroscopist sits, and assistant stabilizes patient's knee so that it does not roll externally.

Anteromedial compartment

Complete inspection of the anteromedial compartment may be facilitated by redirection of the endoscope. From initial placement 30° laterally, the scope is removed and the blunt trocar is reinserted and directed toward the medial meniscus.

The physician stands up and applies valgus strain to the patient's knee while the assistant provides support to the lateral femur (Fig. 3-22). With internal and external rotation of the tibia and with flexion and extension, and excellent composite of the medial compartment can be recorded. In most patients, it is possible to pass under the meniscus with a 1.7-mm diameter Needlescope. Horizontal cleft tears back to the area of the coronary ligament attachment can be inspected. In some patients acute coronary ligament tears have been identified. Examination proceeds from the anterior portion of the posterior horn to the meniscus and its medial substance and then to the anterior horn; a return to the medial substance and up the meniscal surface to the meniscal-synovial junction completes the procedure. In this area, the endoscope can be passed forward, adjacent to the attachment to the tibial collateral ligament (see Fig. 9-1, *H* and *J*). If an area with no definition is found ("white out") I recommend moving back to the horizon of the femoral condyle to reestablish location and then proceeding to the unknown areas. Flexion and extension can demonstrate mobility of the meniscus and can improve viewing of any particular area; in fact, it is possible to follow the tangent of the medial femoral condyle all the way into the suprapatellar pouch for complete examination. It is not unusual with stress on the knee to see a serpentine border on the inner portion of the meniscus (see Fig. 7-1, *D*). Findings of the condylar surface should be recorded.

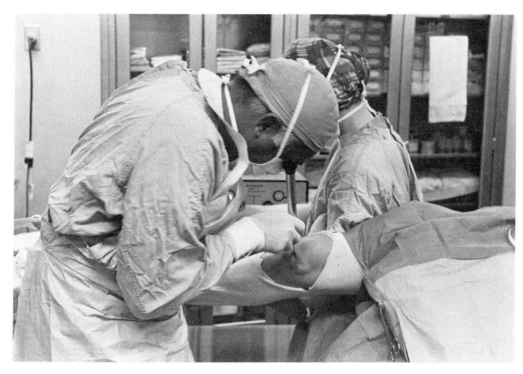

FIG. 3-22. Inspection of anteromedial compartment is facilitated by nurse placing her elbow and body against distal lateral femur and arthroscopist applying valgus stress to patient's knee. Notice safe distance between arthroscopist's eye and hand, reducing potential for contamination.

Posteromedial compartment

After the anterior compartments have been viewed, the endoscope is removed and the *joint is redistended to maximum* with saline to facilitate the posterior compartment inspection.

The patient's hip is rotated externally and his knee is slightly flexed. The assistant supports the patient's thigh. The physician sits with the patient's foot in his lap (Fig. 3-23).

The area of entry is posterior to the tibial collateral ligament, superior to the meniscus, and posterior to the medial femoral condyle. In thin patients it is possible to see a bulge in this area when the knee is distended. The cannula and sharp trocar are directed parallel to the tibial condyles and directly into the posterior compartment (Fig. 3-24). With removal of the sharp trocar, extravasation of saline confirms the entry (Fig. 3-25), and visualization is then possible. The landmark for orientation is the junction between the meniscus and the femoral condyle, and with advancement of the endoscope it is possible in many patients to see the posterior cruciate ligament (see Fig. 7-8, *A* and *B*). Inspection down the posterior aspect of the meniscus will show any vertical rim tears or separation from the attachment. In some patients it is possible to see into a Baker's cyst.

A second position that has proved advantageous is placement of the tibia in marked internal rotation, which drops the meniscus off the femoral condyle. This allows viewing down the superior surface of the medial meniscus, which is not possible anteriorly because the curve of the condyle blocks the view.

On completion of this inspection, the knee is redistended with saline to facilitate entry to the posterolateral compartment.

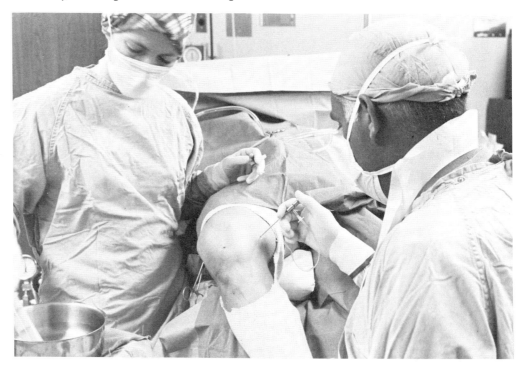

FIG. 3-23. Posteromedial puncture is made with cannula and sharp trocar, parallel to tibial condyles and posterior to meniscus. Arthroscopist can palpate the "soft spot" in maximally distended joint.

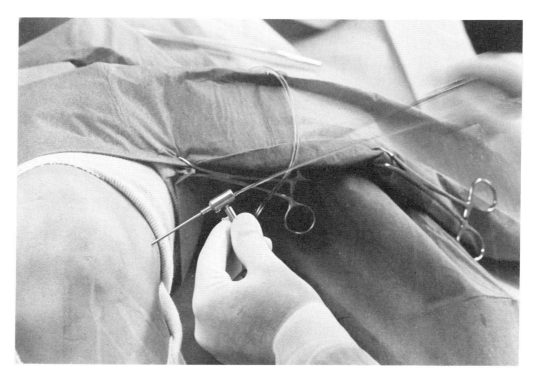

FIG. 3-24. Extrusion of saline from cannula confirms entry of cannula into joint. It is especially important that posteromedial and posterolateral entries be made into maximally distended joint. This facilitates entry and confirms penetration.

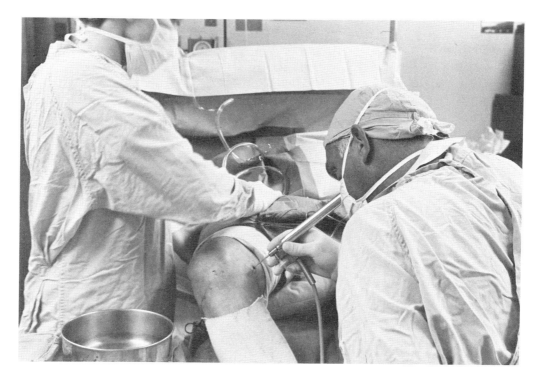

FIG. 3-25. In posteromedial approach, patient's hip is rolled into external rotation and knee is flexed; foot rests in arthroscopist's lap. Thus posteromedial portion of knee joint can be entered with relative ease and freedom.

Posterolateral compartment

The assistant moves to an area next to the patient's pelvis. The patient's hip is moved into adduction, and the knee is flexed approximately 100°. The arthroscopist stands facing the lateral aspect of the patient's thigh. After placing his foot on a stool rung, the surgeon can rest the patient's leg on his thigh (Fig. 3-26). During this repositioning, it is necessary that the circulating nurse move the Mayo stand and the light source to make room for the arthroscopist.

The landmark for the posterolateral puncture is at a point where a line drawn along the lateral intermuscular septum intersects with a second line drawn parallel to the posterior margin of the fibula (Fig. 3-27). At this site the skin is lanced, and a cannula with a sharp trocar is inserted and directed slightly anterior and slightly inferior. With palpation, the instrument is placed in the posterolateral compartment. The previous anteromedial puncture and the distended lateral joint line immediately superior to the meniscus can be helpful in orientation.

Maximum distention of the joint may be compromised by minimal leakage from previous puncture wounds. This can be compensated for by detaching the K-52 catheter from the cannula, attaching it to a No. 18 needle, placing it in the joint anteromedially (this area was anesthetized prior to initial puncture), and reinstilling saline (Fig. 3-28). Extrusion of fluid from the cannula again confirms entry (Fig. 3-29).

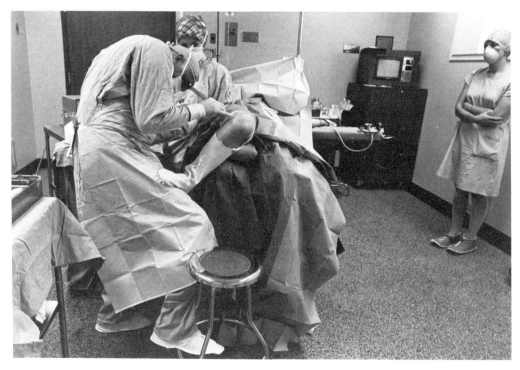

FIG. 3-26. Posterolateral inspection is facilitated by surgeon's placing foot on a stool rung so that patient's foot can rest on thigh. This frees arthroscopist's hands for posterolateral inspection of patient's knee. Mayo stand, light source, and assistant are in more proximal positions.

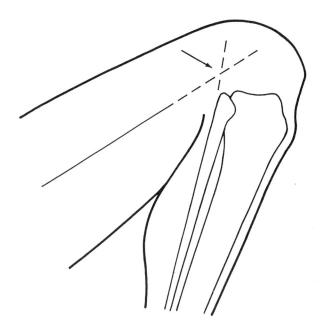

FIG. 3-27. Point of posterolateral entry where line drawn up from lateral intermuscular septum intersects with line drawn up from posterior aspect of fibula. Trocar and sharp cannula are placed, then directed slightly inferior and anterior to enter posterolateral compartment.

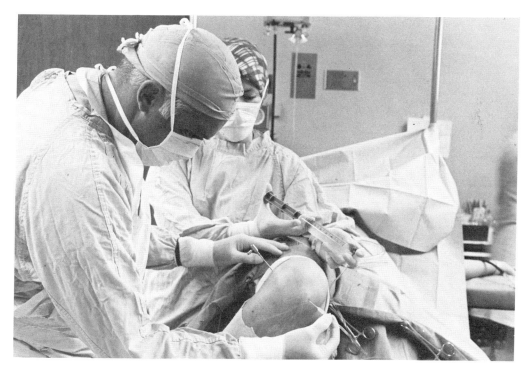

FIG. 3-28. Posterolateral approach is often facilitated by saline forced into joint to create maximal distention. Syringe from polyethylene catheter can be attached to No. 18 needle and placed through the previous anteromedial puncture site.

The internal landmark is the junction of the meniscus and the lateral femoral condyle (Fig. 7-2, *E*). This has a little different contour here than on the medial side. Posterior loose bodies and posterior detached menisci are visible that cannot be seen from other approaches. It has been possible to enter the popliteus sheath in some cases, but in my opinion success was fortuitous. The popliteus sheath under the meniscus often houses loose bodies, which can be vacuumed out at this time.

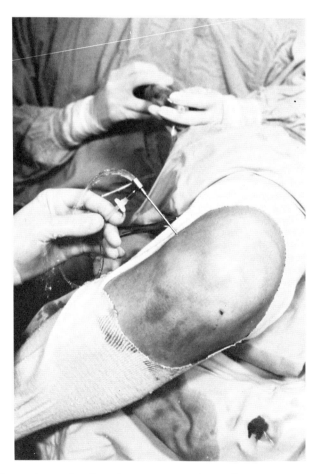

FIG. 3-29. Extrusion of saline from posterolateral puncture confirms entry.

Auxiliary suprapatellar approach

In some situations an auxiliary suprapatellar puncture is indicated. This is most easily performed with the patient's leg extended and the physician sitting medial to the knee, while the assistant stabilizes the thigh to the outer side (Fig. 3-30). The point of entry is at the level of the superior margin of the patella and ³⁄₄ inch below the surface of the knee. The direction is perpendicular to the long axis of the leg and parallel to the floor. Upon entry it is possible to see the undersurface of the patella (see Fig. 10-1, *B*). Articular surface visualization is facilitated by manipulation of the patella. The intercondylar notch and the fat pad can be seen, as well as any loose bodies in the suprapatellar pouch.

In patients who have suspected subluxation or dislocation of the patella, a lateral suprapatellar inspection is indicated. The patient's leg is extended, and the physician and the assistant change places so that the physician is on the outer aspect of the knee. The puncture site and technique are similar to those of medial entry, allowing visualization of the defect in the lateral femoral condyle. A loose body may be engulfed in the synovium along the lateral femoral condyle (see Fig. 10-1, *E*).

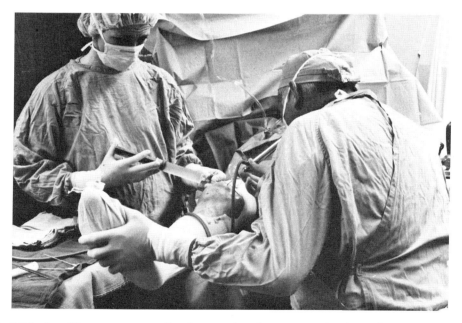

FIG. 3-30. Auxiliary suprapatellar inspection is commonly done from medial side at level of superior aspect of patella. If acute dislocation of patella is suspected, lateral inspection is indicated. This allows visualization down lateral sulcus for any potential loose bodies and also may allow defect in lateral femoral condyle to be seen.

FOLLOW-UP

After an arthroscopic examination with local anesthesia, a simple compression bandage is applied to the puncture sites (Figs. 3-31 and 3-32). The patient is advised to remove this dressing the following day and to place Band-Aids over the small wounds. Because patients frequently forget what they have been told in the operating room, the following week in the office their puncture wounds are inspected and the arthroscopic findings are reviewed.

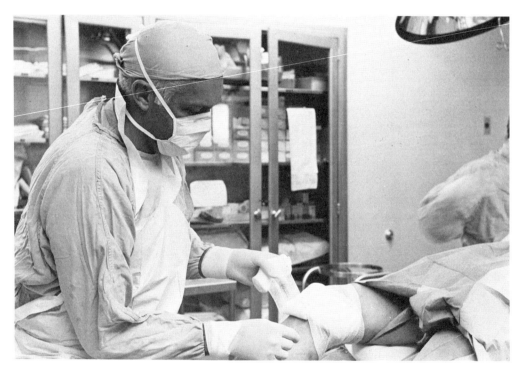

FIG. 3-31. After arthroscopic procedure, gauze bandages are placed over small puncture wounds and sterile dressing compresses joint. Next day, patient may remove bandage and place small Band-Aids over areas of entry.

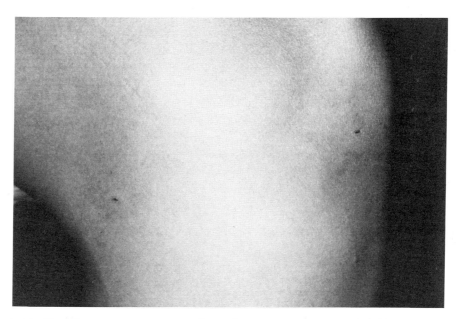

FIG. 3-32. Needlescope leaves small marks, seen here 1 week following multiple-puncture technique arthroscopy. Punctures are so small that no suture is required, and Band-Aid is all that is indicated after second day. Surgery can be performed any day after arthroscopy without risk of infection.

COMPLICATIONS

In two patients the saphenous vein was nicked with a No. 11 blade while making the posteromedial puncture. One patient bled for 3 days despite application of a compression dressing. The bleeding subsided spontaneously, and there was no further complication. The other patient underwent arthrotomy while under general anesthesia. Although the vein was ligated, there was no subsequent complication of phlebitis.

There has been no infection or unexplained synovitis as a result of arthroscopy. A few patients have developed synovial inflammation following surgery, but neither anaerobic nor aerobic culture tests showed any positive results. There were no wound infections following any arthroscopy in the past 4 years.

One patient who had a Waldeus total-knee prosthesis with absorption adjacent to the cement line underwent arthroscopy, at which time it was determined that he had a preexistent low-grade infection. The hemarthrosis produced during arthroscopy created a culture medium for the bacteria, and subsequent drainage of the knee and removal of the prosthesis were necessitated. However, we have performed arthroscopies on patients who had acutely infected knees, without any exacerbation of the condition or puncture-site infection.

In one patient synovial fluid drained for 4 days after a loose body of 1-inch diameter was removed percutaneously from the posteromedial compartment with a Jaws modified pituitary ronjeur during arthroscopy. No sutures were placed in the synovium or skin of this patient, in whom a skin incision of approximately 1 cm had been made. The problem cleared without sequelae.

REFERENCES

1. Burman, M. S., Finkelstein, H., and Mayer, L.: Arthroscopy of the knee joint, J. Bone Joint Surg. **16:**255-268, 1934.
2. Guten, G. N.: Methylene blue staining of articular cartilage during arthroscopy, Orthop. Rev. **6:**59-60, 1977.
3. Jackson, R. W., and Abe, I.: The role of arthroscopy in the management of disorders of the knee; an analysis of 200 consecutive examinations, J. Bone Joint Surg. **54:**310-322, 1972.

Chapter 4

Anesthesia

LOCAL ANESTHESIA

On October 30, 1972, I performed my first arthroscopy, without having witnessed one. The lack of experience proved to be advantageous in developing the technique of knee joint arthroscopy with the patient under local anesthesia. I am not aware of any previous reports of a technique with local anesthetic.

In the first patients, only 1% lidocaine was administered, into the skin, subcutaneous tissue, and the synovium; no intra-articular tissue was anesthetized. Successful visualization of the anterior and superior compartments of the joint was accomplished. Subsequently it was realized that if the infrapatellar branch of the saphenous nerve were blocked, there was a decrease in the patient's sense of proprioception, and improved relaxation resulted (Fig. 4-1).

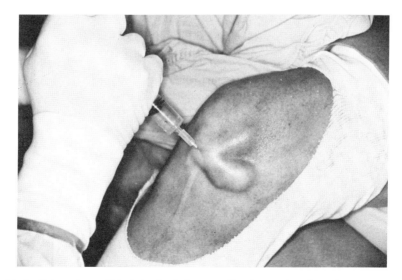

FIG. 4-1. Plain lidocaine, 1%, blocks infrapatellar branch of saphenous nerve. This decreases patient's sense of proprioception and anxiety and increases comfort during procedure.

Initially, a narcotic or sedative was given intravenously. Patients often became drowsy and occasionally nauseated, and they frequently vomited. The use of such medicine prolonged the outpatient stay in the recovery room. Also, patients were restricted from driving vehicles. Therefore, this practice was stopped, and subsequent experience has shown it to be unnecessary.

Technique

After it has been established medically that arthroscopy is indicated, the patient is given the choice of having it performed with local anesthetic. Most patients readily accept this because of the simplicity and reduced risk of the procedure.

Plain lidocaine, 1%, is used. It has not been necessary to inject local anesthetic inside the joint cavity, because an adequate infiltrative block of the infrapatellar fat pad and the infrapatellar branch of the saphenous nerve has sufficed for inspection of the anterior and superior compartments. For posteromedial, posterolateral, and auxillary suprapatellar punctures, direct locally infiltrated 1% plain lidocaine is injected (Fig. 4-2). Normally, 10 to 12 ml of lidocaine are used per puncture, but a higher dose is indicated in a sensitive person.

It is essential that the patient not be hurt or punished. A dialogue between the surgeon and the patient can avoid this; if there is any discomfort, the patient should speak up. If the cannula and trocar are in place when the discomfort occurs, remove the trocar, bend the K-52 catheter at the entry site, and place lidocaine through the cannula to that exact area (Fig. 4-3). This delivers the anesthetic better than does withdrawing the cannula or trying to pass a needle adjacent to the cannula to achieve adequate anesthesia in the area.

There are several other factors that facilitate arthroscopy when the patient is under local anesthesia. First and perhaps foremost is the security and confidence of the arthroscopist, whose attitude is readily perceived by the patient. Confidence transmitted to the patient will result in relaxation and decreased anxiety. Second, a gentle procedure carried out with dispatch (less than 15 minutes) is easily tolerated. Third, the patient's confidence and relaxation can be enhanced by word-of-mouth advertising by other patients who had successful arthroscopies.

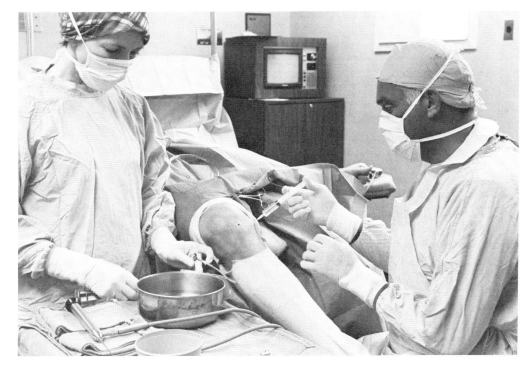

FIG. 4-2. Plain lidocaine, 1%, is injected directly into posteromedial compartment. Direct infiltration is also utilized in posterolateral approach.

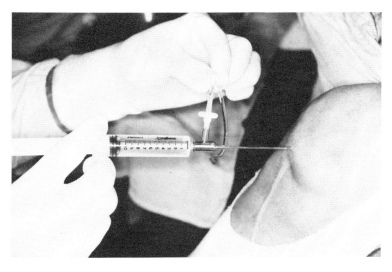

FIG. 4-3. If patient expresses some discomfort during insertion of scope, rather than withdraw cannula and reinsert needle, it is possible to pinch off K-52 catheter and infiltrate 1% plain lidocaine directly through cannula to tip, exact site where patient is having discomfort.

Patient instruction

The physician should inform the patient of the nature of the arthroscopic procedure. One of the most valuable methods of allaying anxiety and fear is to give the patient a mimeographed instruction sheet about arthroscopy (see box below). First reading may create some anxiety, but at the time of the procedure, the patient may find that it has been of considerable comfort in reducing his apprehension. He will be pleased to find that the procedure is carried out as detailed.

After the procedure, a dressing is applied (see Fig. 3-32); it is removed the following day, and Band-Aids are placed over the multiple puncture wounds. If there

---

ARTHROSCOPY INSTRUCTIONS

Arthroscopy (looking into a joint) is a relatively new procedure, now performed with a fiberoptic Needlescope of small diameter (2.2 mm). It takes about 10 minutes.

Arthroscopy allows the physician to directly visualize most every portion of the knee joint and provides an opportunity to improve diagnostic accuracy. The intended purpose is to prevent unnecessary surgery and dictate earlier surgical intervention in those patients requiring an operation.

The procedure is performed in the hospital outpatient operating room so as to provide ideal conditions. The procedure necessitates the use of a tourniquet (a tight tube) placed around your thigh to prevent any small amount of blood from obscuring the physician's vision. This tourniquet tightness is the most uncomfortable part of the procedure. If you remain relaxed and do not tighten up, the tourniquet will be more tolerable. Your leg is painted with a cool, brown antiseptic solution. Sterile sheets protect the area. Your knees will be allowed to bend so your legs hang down.

You will have some discomfort with the "freezing" of the knee, which is similar to that done by a dentist. The medicine is 1% lidocaine and usually renders the knee painless. There may be a feeling of distention or occasional pressure without pain.

There are complications to any procedure, and so it is with arthroscopy. There is less than 1% chance of complication. The known problems have been breakage of the fiberoptic scope, infection, allergy to the medicines used, and knee effusion (swelling). These are rare, and we take measures to prevent them.

Now for your part:
1. You will be called by the hospital regarding your time of arrival.
2. Please shave your leg (groin to ankle) and shower prior to the test.
3. Bring a list of any known allergies to medicines and/or general medical problems for our information.
4. Anticipate 1 to 2 hours total time to get in and out of the hospital.

Thank you.

is no indication for surgical intervention, the patient is examined approximately 1 week following the arthroscopic examination, and the arthroscopic findings are reviewed at that time. If the patient is scheduled for surgery, this review will be carried out the night prior to surgery. Surgery can safely be performed immediately, a day, or a week after Needlescope arthroscopy, without an increased risk of infection.

I have performed these as early as 1 day and as late as 10 or more days after arthroscopy for 4 years, with no patient developing infection of the small (2 mm) arthroscopic puncture wounds. In an occasional case contamination has required redraping and repreparing the patient. Although with the Needlescope the eyepiece is at a safe distance from the surgeon's hand, when using an arthroscope in which the ocular lens is close to the hand the chance of contamination is great, and it is safer to reprepare and redrape the patient prior to arthrotomy.

Patient selection

The selection of patients for arthroscopic examination under local anesthesia is based on clinical judgment. If the patient has a diagnostic problem without clear-cut physical findings to support complaints, then arthroscopy is performed with local anesthetic. To be more specific, preoperative assessment is important in advising a patient who has had many previous surgeries. It affords an opportunity to discuss with the patient the arthroscopic findings, prospective surgery, and prognosis. Both the surgeon and the patient have increased confidence when a surgical procedure can be designed after direct observation of intra-articular findings.

Patients whose history and physical examination suggest a meniscal abnormality, but in whom positive findings are lacking, are also given arthroscopy with local anesthetic. If physical examination is compromised because the patient has pain, diagnosis may be established by arthroscopy rather than by surgical exploration. This not only avoids the risk of general anesthetic, but also eliminates unnecessary arthrotomy or meniscectomy. Misdiagnosis of patellar conditions (i.e., chondromalacia, dislocation, or subluxation) can be avoided. In some patients with condylar disease (i.e., osteochondritis dissecans), the status of the articular surface cannot be demonstrated on arthrogram or plain-film roentgenogram; arthroscopy can provide this information. Ligamentous injuries, both fresh and old, are amenable to arthroscopic examination. Synovial disease also lends itself to morphologic study by this technique.

Recent series have included a number of patients with medicolegal or Workmen's Compensation claims, who were seen for evaluation only. In the minds of the referring physicians, these patients probably had no knee problem, and the consultation was to confirm that impression. Although we would like to think of arthroscopy as contributing in a positive way, these examinations performed for purposes of ruling out any existing abnormality allow the physician to proceed with confidence in recommending conservative measures.

Patient monitoring

The arthroscopist can anticipate any sudden moves by the patient by being sensitive to his reactions. During the procedure with local anesthesia, the arthroscopist can monitor the patient's discomfort or anxiety by observing his breathing or deep sighing. The patient will tighten his Achilles tendon, which can be monitored easily by the surgeon, whose hand is on the patient's ankle (see Fig. 3-10). It should also be noted that when a patient under local anesthesia tightens his quadriceps muscle, the capsular tissues will be compressed, making it difficult to puncture the fascia.

Discussion

When the technical principles previously outlined are carefully adhered to, it is possible to arthroscopically examine the entire knee joint with the patient under local anesthesia.

The value of local anesthesia cannot be overemphasized. With essentially no risk to the patient, a comprehensive evaluation of the diagnostic problem is possible, as are some therapeutic measures (i.e., removal of loose bodies). The patient's pain threshold and psychologic sensitivity to the knee problem can be evaluated during injection of the local anesthetic. Areas within the knee can be palpated to confirm the presence of an intra-articular abnormality.

As with any surgical procedure, there is no substitute for sound clinical judgment, knowledge of anatomy, preparation and organization, and perseverence in improving clinical skills through experience.

Tourniquet. The use of the tourniquet has been questioned. However, arthroscopy can be performed in 5 to 15 minutes, and the patient is able to tolerate the tightness on the thigh for this period of time. In fact, there is some anesthetic effect from ischemia. Inspection of the joint can be bloodless. At the end of the procedure, the tourniquet is released and the vascular characteristics of the synovium are documented.

Physician-patient relationship. Do not underestimate the effect of verbal and written explanation given to the patient in order to allay his anxiety. An existing physician-patient relationship has proved to be important in establishing relaxation. Some of the more difficult patients have been those who were referred for arthroscopic examination only.

Diagnostic value. Arthroscopy with local anesthetic was performed on patients in whom circumstantial evidence (i.e., history and physical examination, roentgenograms, and arthrogram) was not sufficient to warrant surgical exploration or on patients referred for evaluation only. Without arthroscopy, certain of these patients would have undergone empirical exploratory arthrotomy; others would have been treated conservatively. The matching of the right treatment to the right condition in this group of patients would have been a matter of chance. Arthroscopy with local anesthetic provided a method of reaching a correct diagnosis by direct evidence and hence of prescribing the appropriate treatment.

GENERAL ANESTHESIA
Technique

The technique of arthroscopy is the same when performed with the patient under general anesthesia. Posteromedial and posterolateral inspections are still important in any patient in whom inspection from the anterior puncture shows normal findings, because of the possibility of lesions not seen from other approaches.

The patient's position is the same for arthroscopy as for arthrotomy. At the end of the arthroscopic procedure, the equipment and its tables are moved away, and separate Mayo stands and tables for the arthrotomy are positioned. A new water-impermeable drape is placed on the table.

Arthroscopy has not lengthened the duration of general anesthesia, but actually shortens the procedure time. The inspection of the knee by arthroscopy is thorough; thus extensive surgical exploration and unnecessary arthrotomies are avoided. It is possible to make selective and rather limited incisions because of the knowledge of the intra-articular lesion gained by arthroscopy. A time limit of 15 minutes for arthroscopy should be established, so as to not discourage the operating team. With experience, arthroscopy is not a hindrance to the operating schedule but is of benefit to both the surgeon and the anesthesiologist.

Patient selection

Arthroscopy with general anesthetic is performed on patients who have not had a recent arthroscopy of the knee with local anesthetic but whose known clinical condition warrants surgical intervention.

A small percentage of patients who would be candidates for arthroscopy with local anesthetic for diagnostic purposes choose or are advised to have arthroscopy with general anesthetic because of personal or emotional reasons. This might include those patients who have had multiple arthroscopies, done either to follow a defect in the articular cartilage or because of subsequent injury to the knee. Only one of my patients experienced enough discomfort during the initial procedure with local anesthetic that he requested that the second be done with general anesthetic. Most patients, when given the choice, choose a local anesthetic if there is some certainty that an arthrotomy will not follow.

COMPLICATIONS

We have seen no complications from anesthetic in arthroscopy. No patients have shown sensitivity to 1% plain lidocaine, and none have developed pulmonary emboli or thrombophlebitis, even with an accompanying arthrotomy. It should be noted that patients 40 or more years of age who had arthrotomies were given low-dosage prophylactic warfarin sodium (Coumadin).

REFERENCES

1. Johnson, L. L.: Arthroscopy of the knee using local anesthesia: a review of 400 patients, J. Bone Joint Surg. (Am.) **58**(5):736,1976.
2. Johnson, L. L. Diagnostic arthroscopy of the knee: the knee joint. Amsterdam, Excerpta Medica; New York, 1974, American Elsevier Publishing Co., pg. 131-319, 1974.

Chapter 5

Impact of arthroscopy
on clinical practice

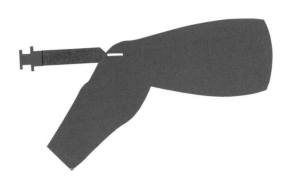

Arthroscopy has sparked the curiosity and interest of most orthopedists. Heretofore the technique with large-diameter endoscopes and general anesthetic, confining the inspection to the anterior portion of the knee joint, was not considered practical and thus was not embraced as part of routine management in orthopedics.

When the concept of arthroscopy was expanded to include the use of local anesthetic and inspection of posteromedial and posterolateral compartments, arthroscopy became a valuable necessity.

Still some orthopedists vehemently reject the value of arthroscopy. It seems to challenge the competence and clinical abilities of some; others admit inability to technically perform the procedure with proficiency. This is in sharp contrast to the widespread acceptance by patients with knee problems who have come to understand the value of arthroscopy. Patients who realize that the interior of the joint can be inspected directly under local anesthesia will choose arthroscopy over an exploratory arthrotomy, regardless of the confidence they or the surgeon might have in the clinical evaluation.

Because proficiency in arthroscopy points up limitations of clinical diagnosis and lack of understanding of pathologic processes in patients with knee problems, orthopedists who have invested time, money, and energy in arthroscopy have been rewarded handsomely by improvement of diagnostic skills, understanding of pathologic findings, and general enjoyment of their practice. Those who have not expended the energy to become proficient in arthroscopy cannot make a valid criticism and simply do not know what they are missing.

ENHANCEMENT OF CLINICAL SKILLS

Interest in arthroscopy and its benefits does not negate the physician's desire to improve other clinical skills of physical examination, laboratory testing, or x-ray film interpretation. It provides further information on which to evaluate clinical judgment and diagnostic competence. A continued reshaping of clinical impressions is possible. For instance, during clinical review (documented later in this chapter) it was not unusual to find that either an additional significant or different diagnosis than that made preoperatively was identified by arthroscopy. Also, in a few patients complete arthroscopic examination of the joint proved that no abnormality existed, although clinical, laboratory, or x-ray findings suggested one.

Certain conditions may be clinically suspected but confirmed by arthroscopy only. For example, subluxation of the patella may be a subtle condition. It can be overlooked clinically, but the specific lesion is seen arthroscopically in the lateral femoral condyle.

Correlation of clinical experience with arthroscopic findings increases the physician's confidence in caring for patients with knee problems, which certainly enhances the enjoyment of practice for the orthopedist/arthroscopist.

EFFECT ON PATIENT MANAGEMENT

A patient's symptoms, physical signs, and x-ray findings provide information on which the clinician may base one of three choices: conservative management (i.e., laboratory investigation, medication, or exercises); arthroscopic examination with local anesthetic for those patients in whom diagnosis is uncertain; or surgical intervention based on recognition of typical findings of an internal derangement or other surgically amenable abnormalities. Many patients will require arthroscopic evaluation if other attempts at diagnosis fail or they are unimproved after conservative treatment.

Over the past several years, the management of acute knee injuries has evolved from a concept of "wait and see" to one of earlier definitive treatment. Evaluation of any instability clinically or arthrographic evidence of intra-articular abnormalities is being substituted. The "wait and see" attitude really is "not seeing at all;" it is postponing treatment to a time when surgical repair might be compromised or the intra-articular injury may be permanent. This is compounded if the patient attempts to mobilize a knee with internal derangement.

Therefore arthroscopy has replaced the "wait and see" method with the "see" method. The aspiration of hemarthrosis, followed by roentgenography to rule out fracture and the subsequent application of a cast, is probably no longer generally accepted practice. Hemarthrosis is not considered a contraindication to arthroscopy. By the methods outlined in previous chapters, clear visualization can be achieved intra-articularly in the acutely injured knee. Therefore, there is very little excuse for a delay in arthroscopy, resultant diagnosis, and treatment.

For example, a massive hemarthrosis may accompany a torn anterior cruciate ligament, a complete separation of a posteromedial meniscus, or an acute dislocation of the patella. The patient's acute pain may compromise the clinical examination, and in the presence of hemarthrosis, the arthrogram loses its reliability. An arthroscopic examination provides an immediate definitive diagnosis. Appropriate early treatment is pursued with confidence.

Arthroscopy provides a means of differential diagnosis and direction in patient management. It allows a macroscopic inspection of the joint previously possible only by arthrotomy. Because fluid is instilled in the joint, the natural activities of flexion, extension, and rotation can be simulated during arthroscopic observation. This enhances recognition of various pathologic abnormalities. The subtle early degenerative changes not recognized grossly are readily apparent arthroscopically.

DIFFERENTIAL DIAGNOSIS

Many patients when seen clinically have symptoms suggesting intra-articular abnormalities, but no positive physical, laboratory, or x-ray findings. They desire a definitive determination of the problem and some clear-cut direction for treatment. In the past such patients were advised to pursue conservative measures until the condition resolved through the natural course or worsened to such an extent that diagnosis was obvious. Even exploratory surgery may be acceptable to the patient if it is the only viable alternative to symptoms.

In contrast, arthroscopy provides a method of inspecting the interior of the joint completely to establish or rule out intra-articular abnormalities. The physician can then institute appropriate intervention or conservative measures based on this observation.

Arthroscopy provides understanding of management in vague diagnoses. Often patients have vague complaints referable to their knees, but no sign of intra-articular abnormality. Typically, there is tenderness along the medial joint line, pain in the patellar area with some minimal patellar catching, or crepitus that is barely discernible. If symptoms are caused by chondromalacia of the patella, the physician can assure the patient that the natural history of this condition rarely produces serious consequences and that conservative isometric exercises and salicylates are indicated. On the other hand, if a torn meniscus is injuring the articular cartilage, the treatment of choice is meniscectomy at an early date, before deterioration of the condylar surfaces results in permanent condylar injury.

A better understanding of the pathologic variations is possible when the arthroscopist correlates results of physical examination with intra-articular observations. Arthroscopic examination of the meniscal dynamics has shown that some menisci are more mobile than others. Certainly if there is no injury to the articular cartilage, the increased mobility of the meniscus need not be treated. However, if there is instability during high-level athletic performance, and if the patient understands the consequences, a meniscectomy might be indicated. Observations of "hypermobile meniscus" made arthroscopically have prevented unnecessary meniscectomy.

ARTHROSCOPY VERSUS ARTHROGRAPHY

Arthroscopy provides a diagnostic bridge between arthrography and subsequent surgical management. X-ray films provide only shadows for interpretation. At best, this is circumstantial evidence. The interpretation of lateral meniscal lesions by arthrography is difficult in the best of hands. Articular and synovial lesions usually are not recognized. A complete absence of the anterior cruciate ligament may be identified arthrographically, but is also easily diagnosed on physical examination. Arthrography is compromised in the presence of hemarthroses, is of limited value if there are large loose bodies, and is of no value in discerning multiple small loose bodies. Arthrography provides limited information about synovial diseases or their morphologic characteristics.

Proponents of the use of arthrography and arthroscopy usually limit arthroscopic examination to the anterior compartments of the joint and use a large-diameter endoscope. Their judgment to continue using arthrography is clinically justified for the posterior aspects of the joint and menisci. Those areas can be documented arthrographically.

Certainly arthrography has been proved an excellent and reliable diagnostic means by those who regularly examine a large volume of patients. It should be continued accepted practice, especially in areas where there is no one skilled in arthroscopy.

I find the direct evidence provided by arthroscopy in all compartments of the joint preferable to the circumstantial findings of arthrography. At the present time, I use arthrography for those patients who have juxta-articular cysts, in order to establish the extent of the mass prior to resection. Also, arthrography can be utilized if it is felt that the arthroscopic examination had been compromised in some area or compartment of the joint.

EFFECT ON SURGICAL DESIGN

Arthroscopy provides additional information for the surgeon in designing and recommending a plan of treatment. It is not unusual that an anticipated surgical procedure is deemed unnecessary as a result of arthroscopy. With experience, interpretation of findings can rule out the need for exploratory arthrotomy or meniscectomy. In some situations, arthroscopic findings greatly alter the anticipated surgical procedure or the location and extent of the incision necessary to perform the definitive treatment.

Arthroscopy can provide information important to maintaining a good physician-patient relationship in complex situations, such as when a second or third exploratory or reconstructive procedure is necessary. The presence or absence of articular degeneration affects the prognosis and is an important consideration when advising a patient who has had previous surgery and is anticipating another operation. The patient gains added confidence in the recommendation of surgery when he has a clear understanding of the anticipated results and the specific prognosis.

Arthroscopic evaluation may prove beneficial in patients with degenerative articular disease who are being considered for high tibial osteotomy or total-knee replacement. Standing x-ray examinations do not fully disclose the status of the articular cartilage or loose bodies in lateral compartments. Tibial osteotomy, which shifts weight bearing to a compartment with significant articular surface loss or meniscal derangement, should be avoided, if possible. Patient selection and surgical results should improve treatment.

REHABILITATION

Rehabilitation is faster as a result of arthroscopy. Significant abnormalities are not overlooked at the time of surgery, such as conditions in the posterior compartment, which if not recognized and treated properly would prolong or complicate the postoperative course. Loose bodies in the posterior compartment that are not visible anteriorly may be removed arthroscopically, thus avoiding prolonged synovitis that would develop while this articular material was absorbed by the synovium. Virtually every recess of the knee joint can be examined and loose articular debris cleared.

Subtle lesions, such as horizontal cleft tears, can be seen with a small-diameter endoscope passing under the meniscus. In addition, posterior horn tears not visualized even from anterior arthrotomy can be seen by posterior arthroscopic examination. When these are observed prior to the initial surgery, they can be surgically managed, removing any potential cause of postoperative problems.

Patients who have recently undergone major reconstructive knee surgery and have articular changes either accompanying or following surgery may benefit by arthroscopy.

After meniscectomy, an occasional patient will have recurring meniscal symptoms or persistent effusion. Prior to arthroscopy with local anesthetic, these patients could only be encouraged to alternately rest and lift weight. Now if there is any unexplained morbidity 8 to 12 weeks after meniscectomy, a direct inspection should be considered. While this may seem an oversell of arthroscopy, my observations have shown this not to be so. The procedure has shown tears of the meniscus in the opposite compartment not present at the time of the original surgery, presence of rather large loose bodies, and an occasional diffuse reactive synovitis. Also, two bucket-handle tears of the regenerated meniscus have been seen.

The presence of loose bodies is the most common cause of effusion following meniscectomy. A preexisting articular injury may flake off more material. Arthroscopy can confirm this, and the material can be removed through the various arthroscopic cannulas. One of the most common causes of postoperative effusions and loose bodies is excessive progressive quadriceps exercises before healing of the surgical incision. The existence of diffuse synovitis will respond to arthroscopic cleansing of fibrin, free synovial debris, and a single injection of cortisone. Removal will interrupt the naturally slow rehabilitative process. The patient will regain muscular strength faster and can resume activity sooner. When the inflammation and thickness about a joint is removed, the patient's confidence in arthroscopy is increased.

RESEARCH

Investigational uses of arthroscopy are limitless now that it can be performed with ease with the patient under local anesthesia. Naturally, patients are hesitant to agree to an exploratory arthrotomy for observation purposes. Some with osteochondritis dissecans, articular defects, or synovial abnormalities have agreed to direct arthroscopic observation. This has not only assisted in treatment of the patient, but has provided increased learning experience for the orthopedist. It has been possible to observe the natural history of osteochondritis dissecans. Direct evidence has been provided as to the extent to which the articular cartilage has loosened and the proper form of treatment.

Healing articular defects are amenable to arthroscopic monitoring. The study of these defects at intervals may influence the advisability and timing of weight bearing. The observations of various methods of treatment of these defects have been documented. Time and experience should establish the value of drilling, curettage, and shaving of articular cartilage. Already we know that drilling of fissured articular cartilage allows it to heal similarly to a fracture. A lesion the size of a dime on a condylar surface will heal and be devoid of blood vessels within 6 weeks. A defect the size of a half dollar takes twice as long to develop an avascular fibrocartilage base. No articular defects that have filled up to the level of the original articular surface have been seen. The histologic healing will correlate exactly with remission of inflammatory signs. Documentation of the healing progress of various sized articular defects is easily recorded photographically. Also, biopsy of the various healing stages with small-cup forceps allows insight into the healing of human cartilage defects.

Previously repaired cruciate ligaments have been observed arthroscopically. Often a ligament that is repaired is absorbed, and only a granular synovium spans the area. Ligaments that have been sutured to the femur may have some substance to them, but when the drawer test is performed under direct observation the ligament stretches and has no integrity. This suggests that suturing of the anterior cruciate ligament to the femur is at best a means of internal debridement. Arthroscopy provides an excellent means of documenting the results of this type of anastomosis.

Observations and morphologic variations of synovial disease have been documented. The medical management of rheumatologic conditions can be monitored arthroscopically. Biopsy in synovial diseases is possible. Articular synovial debris can be submitted by cell block for investigational purposes. Articular changes in degenerative arthritis can be monitored. Arthroscopy may be beneficial in determining whether tibial osteotomy or articular resurfacing is necessary.

REVIEW OF ARTHROSCOPIC EXPERIENCE

A review of clinical experience benefits not only the individual but others who are performing the same procedure or caring for a similar pathologic condition.

The following review demonstrates some specific individual weaknesses in clinical judgment, but provides continued conviction that arthroscopy is of value.

In reviewing my arthroscopic series, several questions were asked: What insight was gained about clinical judgments? What erroneous tendencies were there prearthroscopically? Which conditions were frequently over or underdiagnosed? What effects did increased knowledge have on subsequent arthroscopic indications, methods, and techniques? What changes were made in subsequent patient treatment?

Three series, comprising almost 1,000 patients, were reviewed. *Series I* (October 1972 to September 1975) encompasses the first 400 patients (419 knees) treated under local anesthesia for whom comprehensive clinical records were complete. It should be noted that in a few of the early patients in this series arthroscopy was limited to the front of the knee joint. Most of the patients were examined after it was possible to inspect posteromedially. None of the patients had posterolateral inspections.

Series II (September 1975 to September 1976) includes 375 patients (384 knees) examined under local anesthesia. All had the benefit of the fully developed comprehensive arthroscopy of the knee; that is, the posteromedial and posterolateral compartments were examined even when anterior inspection showed normal findings. In Series II more patients had medicolegal or Workmen's Compensation claims. Arthroscopic consultation was for the purpose of supporting the referring physicians's clinical impressions that the knees were normal and to rule out the presence of occult lesions.

Series III (September 1975 to September 1976) includes 150 consecutive patients (162 knees) examined arthroscopically under general anesthesia immediately prior to an anticipated arthrotomy. All were patients from my private practice. A few had medicolegal or Workmen's Compensation claims.

Choice of anesthetic

Local anesthetic was used for those patients in whom the diagnosis was unconfirmed or the extent of injury or status of the disease process was unclear but arthrotomy was not anticipated. It was also used for those patients in whom the diagnosis seemed certain but for whom a general anesthetic for arthroscopy or arthrotomy was not indicated clinically because they had been referred for consultative arthroscopy only. These patients made up Series I and II.

General anesthetic was used for patients whose history, physical examination, or x-ray findings showed intra-articular lesions or internal derangement that necessitated arthrotomy. Arthroscopy was performed immediately prior to surgery. Series III comprised this group of patients.

Classification of patients

Patients were classified according to five diagnostic categories: meniscal lesions, patellar conditions, condylar disease, extrasynovial lesions, and synovial disease. A miscellaneous category included those patients who were undergoing arthroscopy for medicolegal or consultation purposes.

Patients who had typical symptoms referred to the medial joint line but no positive findings were classified as having a torn medial meniscus. If their symptoms were referred to the lateral joint line, they were placed in the torn lateral meniscus category. Those in the retained posterior meniscus category had had previous arthrotomies through a short anterior incision.

Patients were placed in the patellar or condylar disease categories if the typical history, physical examination, and x-ray evidence suggested those anatomic areas as the most likely sources of their symptoms.

In the extrasynovial disease category were those patients in whom ligamentous injuries, cystic changes, or juxta-articular bony abnormalities were anticipated. In the synovial disease category, patients, typical histories and physical evidence suggested that symptoms were produced in the synovium.

Analysis

Findings of each arthroscopic examination were documented by narrative dictation, drawings in selected cases, or cinephotography in illustrative lesions.

64

Presumptive, or prearthroscopic, diagnosis was compared with the actual arthroscopic findings. Diagnosis was considered correct if confirmed arthroscopically or an additional significant diagnosis was made; it was deemed incorrect if a different diagnosis or no diagnosis was made by arthroscopy. Critical analysis of pre- and postarthroscopic diagnoses provided information on which clinical impressions have been altered over the past several years.

With the prearthroscopic diagnosis in mind, it was determined on the basis of arthroscopic findings whether a lesion was surgically correctable, could be arthroscopically managed, or needed only conservative treatment. No determination was made for arthroscopic examinations carried out for diagnostic purposes only.

Specific analyses of the three series, under each of the five disease categories, are considered in the following sections and in Tables 1 to 10 in the Appendix to this chapter.

Series I

Series I consisted of patients routinely seen in an active private practice. Very few had medicolegal or Workmen's Compensation claims or were referred for diagnostic or second-opinion purposes.

There were 259 male (64%) and 141 female (36%) patients, ranging in age from 8 to 61 years (median, 28 years). Right and left knees were equally represented.

Patients early in this series were examined only in the anterior compartments and the suprapatellar pouch. Subsequently the technique of posteromedial inspection was developed.

Meniscal disease. Initial review showed a considerable tendency prearthroscopically to overdiagnose torn medial menisci. They constituted almost half of the prearthroscopic diagnoses. In part this reflects the frequency of this particular abnormality and the fact that symptoms in many knee conditions are clinically referable to the medial joint line.

Review of postoperative diagnoses shows that the diagnosis of a torn medial meniscus was correct in 24% of patients; a different diagnosis was confirmed in 40%; and no diagnosis was made in 24%, undoubtedly because posteromedial and posterolateral inspections were not carried out in Series I. Common different diagnoses were chondromalacia patellae, degenerative meniscal disease without a tear, or degenerative condylar disease. Eight patients in this group had a torn anterior cruciate ligament without a meniscal abnormality visible from the front. Findings in Series II and III, which included posterior inspection of all knees, suggest that posterior abnormalities in the presence of torn anterior cruciates were probably overlooked in Series I.

Clinical judgment was slightly better in diagnosis of a torn lateral meniscus in patients with symptoms but no clear positive physical or laboratory findings. Diagnosis was confirmed in nine patients (31%). Two patients had a tear of the lateral meniscus plus an old unrepairable tear of the anterior cruciate ligament. In 41% of the patients, a different diagnosis was made, most commonly degeneration of the lateral meniscus or degeneration of the compartment with loose bodies. No diagnosis was made in 20% of patients. This figure is artificially high because no posterolateral punctures were made.

In 28 patients (29 knees), a prearthroscopic diagnosis of retained posterior horn was considered. These patients had had previous surgery carried out through a single short anterior incision. The retained posterior meniscus is commonplace after this type of meniscal arthrotomy, which it is hoped will be eliminated as a standard method of treatment. Suspected retained posterior horn was substantiated arthroscopically in over 90% of the patients. In only two patients was a different diagnosis made; one had a torn lateral meniscus, and the other had a dislocated patella. Arthroscopic findings in patients who have had meniscectomies carried out through a single anterior vertical arthrotomy convinced me of the necessity for removal of the entire meniscus through combined anterior and posterior incisions on the medial side.

Of all meniscal lesions, 38% were surgically correctable, 3% were arthroscopically managed, and 56% were conservatively managed; 3% were diagnosed only (miscellaneous cases). It is significant that more than half of the patients with a torn medial meniscus required only conservative treatment.

In patients with a presumptive diagnosis of a torn lateral meniscus, the arthroscopic examination identified a lesion that was surgically correctable in 37%; 62% were managed conservatively.

In presumptive diagnosis of reatined posterior horn, arthroscopic examination identified a surgically correctable lesion in 58% of the patients; 6% were treated arthroscopically and 34% were conservatively managed.

Of all patients undergoing arthroscopy for clinically suspected meniscal abnormalities with no good positive findings, the majority required only conservative treatment, although a significant percentage still required surgical intervention. Arthroscopy provided a means of differentiating between these two groups of patients for determination of appropriate therapy.

In summary, more patients were categorized as having meniscal disease than actually had it. This was in part due to the presence of medial symptoms in a variety of abnormalities and to a predilection to assume that medial symptoms are meniscal in origin. Statistically, meniscal abnormalities comprise the largest percentage of knee problems.

No posterior inspections were carried out in this group; thus, the number of "no diagnoses" was high.

Patellar conditions. In patients with knee problems, complaints are frequently localized to the area of the patella. An analysis of prearthroscopic impressions of patellar disease indicates that clinical judgment was correct most of the time; the diagnosis was substantiated in 21 of 37 knees examined. A combination of dislocation or subluxation of the patella and chondromalacia was the prevalent additional diagnosis. Occasionally loose bodies were identified even through the anterior puncture. Parapatellar synovitis was diagnosed in two young women with patellar pain and crepitus on flexion and extension and distal push of the patella against the femur. Clinical inspection showed no articular abnormality. A fringe of synovium about the patella was caught between the patella and the femur, producing the symptoms. Conservative measures were adequate for these patients and for most of those with chondromalacia of the patella.

Condylar disease. Patients with degenerative articular disease were examined for the purpose of evaluating the extent of disease or to determine whether a meniscal mechanical abnormality was the cause or aggravating condition. In a number of patients with osteochondritis dissecans, arthroscopy was performed to determine whether the articular surface was intact and to monitor healing in selected patients. Most young patients with osteochondritis dissecans had no loose articular fragments, and healing was accomplished with cast immobilization. Arthroscopic examination was carried out on a few patients with known loose bodies. Small bodies were removed through cannulas or with a pituitary forceps. Because of the technical problems involved in removal of larger loose bodies with a regular pituitary forceps, the reversed-tooth modified pituitary forceps was developed.

Prearthroscopic diagnoses were correct for all patients with condylar disease. Some additional significant diagnoses included degenerative or torn menisci, accompanying degenerative arthritis, and loose bodies. Loose bodies were invariably accompanied by a torn meniscus or degenerative arthritis.

In the condylar disease group, most patients received conservative treatment, mainly because I was not adept at removing loose bodies with the arthroscope. Some loose bodies, however, were removed arthroscopically. The few surgically correctable lesions were in patients who underwent arthroscopy for a loose body or for drilling in osteochondritis dissecans. In four patients a degenerative torn meniscus that was promoting degeneration of articular carlilage was removed. Overall, 17% of condylar problems were surgically correctable, and 80% were conservatively managed.

Extrasynovial lesions. In those patients with extrasynovial abnormalities, a torn tibial collateral ligament was the most common prearthroscopic diagnosis, followed by torn anterior cruciate ligaments.

The clinical impression was substantiated in virtually every patient. A significant number of patients with ligamentous injuries also had additional diagnoses. It was my impression at the time, before the posterior compartments were being inspected, that a patient could have an "isolated" tear of the anterior cruciate ligament. Also, some significant abnormalities accompanying the torn anterior cruciate ligaments were overlooked.

In 40% of patients with a torn tibial collateral ligament, an additional diagnosis was made, most commonly of a torn medial meniscus. Five of these patients had no palpable defects in the tibial collateral ligament nor gross instability. This encouraged arthroscopic intervention in any patient with a partial tear of the tibial collateral ligament, in order not to mobilize a patient with an unsuspected meniscal abnormality.

Forty-one percent of the patients in this group had surgically correctable lesions.

In patients with meniscal cysts, arthroscopic examination rarely showed a bulge within or any degeneration of the meniscus. Subsequent resection of the cyst down to the meniscus was the best indication of the extent of meniscal destruction. If it was minimal, the meniscus was left in. Some patients developed tears with degeneration within 6 months; others have remained completely asymptomatic. These results do not give any clear-cut direction for the management of cystic changes of the menisci. However, the presence of a cystic meniscus with cystic degeneration down into the meniscal abnormality is an indication for meniscectomy.

I was interested in further analysis of the patients with postarthroscopic diagnosis of a torn cruciate ligament. There were 34 such patients in our series, 25 of whom had been clinically classified in other disease categories. In the group presumed to have a torn medial meniscus, 16 patients had torn anterior cruciate ligaments; in six it accompanied the torn lateral meniscus, and in ten it was an "isolated" lesion. In those patients thought to have a torn lateral meniscus, three had a torn cruciate ligament; two accompanied the tear and one was an "isolated" lesion. When a retained posterior meniscal horn was suspected, without physical evidence of a torn cruciate ligament, two such lesions existed. In the 18 patients with torn tibial collateral ligaments, four had an accompanying torn anterior cruciate ligament to some extent. It must be noted that in these patients with known torn tibial collateral ligaments, surgery was not considered because of the lack of a palpable defect or instability. In those 34 patients in whom a torn anterior cruciate ligament was the final diagnosis, surgery was recommended for 21; only one patient refused.

In those patients who underwent surgery, the repair of the anterior cruciate ligament was possible in only one. It was a fresh tear and technically amenable to repair. The others required a reconstructive procedure of some type because instability existed. This further emphasizes the importance of early diagnosis of acute hemorrhagic knees. Most of these patients were seen at a time when neither their original physician nor I recognized the magnitude of the abnormality.

Review of the anterior cruciate ligament tears shows that these can be occult lesions. Most are not diagnosed initially or suspected at the time of clinical examination in patients with diagnostic problems. This could be because the patient tenses the knee, which limits the physicial examination. Isolated sectioning of the anterior cruciate ligament will not produce gross instability of the knee where there is an intact tibial collateral ligament.

Synovial disease. In those patients with synovial disease, preoperative diagnosis was either known synovitis, on the basis of laboratory work, or differential diagnosis of common lesions. Two patients had a history of foreign bodies in the knee. Arthroscopic examination established the existence of a foreign body and articular cartilage scar in one patient. The other patient had no intra-articular foreign body. Most of the patients in this category had arthroscopy for diagnostic purposes, which proved valuable.

Series II

Approximately half of the patients in Series II were referred by other orthopedists for arthroscopic consultation. A large percentage of the referral patients were considered to have no abnormality, and the arthroscopy was performed to rule out a rare or occult abnormality that may not have been identified. A number of these patients had medicolegal or Workmen's Compensation claims.

Of the 375 patients in Series II, 243 were male and 132 were female. They ranged in age from 9 to 76 years. All were given local anesthetic. All knees were inspected posteromedially and posterolaterally, when indicated.

Meniscal disease. As in Series I, a high percentage of prearthroscopic diagnoses fell in the meniscal category. Statistical analysis of meniscal disease was similar in the two series, although diagnostic abilities had improved with experience and inclusion of the posterior puncture to the routine examination. The apparent lack of statistical improvement was related to patient selection in Series II. Many believed to have no clinical abnormality were placed in the torn meniscus group by the referring physician, which accounts for no diagnosis being made in 30% of patients with a torn medial meniscus. With the addition of posterior compartment inspection, additional diagnoses were identified in 16% of patients and a different diagnosis was made in 23%. In the latter group, differential diagnosis was made between chondromalacia of the patella and meniscal abnormality with minimal positive findings. These patients were arbitrarily placed in the torn meniscus group preoperatively. Arthroscopy usually confirmed chondromalacia patellae.

In those referred patients in whom no abnormality was suspected on the basis of history or physical examination, the clinical impression was usually supported by arthroscopy. Many of these patients had emotional concerns or potential secondary gain. Had they been placed in a separate group, overall diagnostic accuracy would have improved statistically.

A torn medial meniscus was suspected in 115 patients. The diagnosis was confirmed in 36. Of these, an additional significant abnormality was diagnosed in 17 patients: degenerative arthritis in six, torn anterior cruciate in five, tear of the lateral meniscus in three, and torn anterior cruciate ligament and torn lateral meniscus in three.

A different diagnosis was established in 27 patients. Chondromalacia was present in 25. Degenerative arthritis was the second most common different diagnosis in the meniscal compartment, occurring in 10 patients. An isolated torn anterior cruciate ligament was seen in four patients, and a torn lateral meniscus in two. Synovitis was seen in two patients, posterior cruciate ligament tear in one, subluxation of the patella in one, loose bodies in one, and a meniscal cyst in one.

Meniscal symptoms referable to the lateral joint line were seen in 45 patients. Of these, 16 had an isolated tear of the lateral meniscus. Three patients had an additional torn anterior cruciate ligament identified only at arthroscopy. A different diagnosis was established in 18 patients: degenerative meniscal or articular abnormality without a mechanical tear in seven; isolated anterior cruciate ligament tear, usually laying out in the lateral joint line and mimicking a torn meniscus, in three; loose bodies in the posterolateral compartment in two; a torn anterior cruciate ligament and degenerative articular disease in one; and subluxation of the patella in one. Patellar tendon tear, chondromalacia, torn meniscus, and synovitis were each seen once. No diagnosis was made in eight patients, despite inspection of all compartments. This review shows that significant abnormalities, especially torn anterior cruciate ligaments, should be suspected when initial symptoms suggest meniscal disease.

It should be noted that posterior puncture revealed five torn lateral menisci that were not seen from the front and that four additional patients had loose bodies seen only in the posterior compartment.

A retained posterior horn was identified in 21 patients, 17 medially and four laterally. Thirteen of these patients had an additional diagnosis, most commonly degenerative arthritis or torn anterior cruciate ligament. It is significant that six of these patients had a posterior meniscal abnormality identified from the posterior puncture only. Some who had a retained posterior horn that was partially excised had a second old meniscal tear behind the line of resection. Four patients had loose bodies identified only by the posterior puncture.

In the group of patients prearthroscopically thought to have a torn meniscus, 23% had a significant abnormality found only by posteromedial and posterolateral puncture. Of torn medial menisci, 18% were identified by this route, as were 9% of loose bodies. Of those patients with a suspected retained meniscus following previous surgery, 48% had an abnormality identified only by the posteromedial and posterolateral puncture of a meniscal tear.

Review of the meniscal group showed again the surprising number of additional abnormalities identified only arthroscopically, in particular by the posterior inspection. I believe this points to the value of arthroscopy, rather than to lack of clinical expertise.

Patellar conditions. Analysis of patellar abnormalities in this series was similar to Series I, with some differences. Four patients had experienced a direct blow to the patella, which injured the articular surface. Some patients with bipartite patellas that showed no fragmentation at the junction had articular abnormalities different from the original observations. After inspection of several patients with bipartite patellas, it was learned that about half have symptomatic separations very much like a nonunion with articular irregularities at the junction.

The clinical impression was substantiated by the arthroscopic examination in most of the patients with patellar disease. Additional diagnoses included chondromalacia, loose bodies, and subluxations. Most patients with dislocation or subluxation also had loose bodies or chondromalacia. Three patients in whom patellar abnormality was the primary diagnosis also had a torn meniscus. One patient had a torn anterior cruciate ligament accompanying a dislocation. Most loose bodies were from the lateral femoral condyle and rested in the lateral sulcus or in the posterolateral compartment. Most were managed arthroscopically.

The main advantage of arthroscopic examination of patients with patellar problems is that surgery or rehabilitative regimen can be specifically designed.

Condylar disease. The prearthroscopic diagnosis of condylar disease was substantiated in virtually every patient. The additional diagnosis of loose bodies or degenerative changes accompanied the primary diagnosis, and an additional torn meniscus or retained posterior horn was seen in two patients. A different diagnosis was made in two patients: one had loose bodies from osteochondromatosis, the other had severe synovitis with catching and popping in the joint mimicking loose bodies and degenerative changes.

Arthroscopy in condylar diseases can establish the extent of the articular erosion; determine whether there is loss all the way down to raw bone, necessitating surgical articular resurfacing; or whether the underlying cause of articular injury is a mechanically torn meniscus that should be surgically removed. Additionally, diffuse degenerative change with loose bodies can be managed arthroscopically, followed by anti-inflammatory medication and isometric quadriceps exercises. This regimen has rendered many patients virtually asymptomatic who otherwise might have been considered for joint resurfacing or total-knee replacement.

Extrasynovial lesions. Forty-eight patients had extrasynovial lesions, arthroscopically confirmed in most.

A significant number of additional diagnoses were made. Most commonly, a torn anterior cruciate ligament was accompanied by a torn medial meniscus. It should be noted that a torn meniscus was suspected, but the primary abnormality was diagnosed as a torn anterior cruciate ligament with minimal instability. One patient had an acute dislocation of the patella as well.

In patients with old ligamentous instability, whether an isolated cruciate ligament tear or rotary instability, concomitant degenerative arthritis, torn meniscus, or loose body was virtually universal. In patients who had previous arthrotomies and an old tear of the anterior cruciate ligament, the most common accompanying abnormality was a retained posterior horn, with degenerative arthritis and loose bodies. Four patients with an old tear of the anterior cruciate ligament had an unidentified torn meniscus. Identification of these additional abnormalities assisted in planning of reconstructive surgery and advising patients of the expected prognosis.

In patients who had acute injuries to the knee, the diagnosis of a torn tibial collateral or cruciate ligament was usually correct. These were usually accompanied by a torn meniscus, either medially or laterally.

Torn tibial collateral ligaments were accompanied by tenderness without gross instability or a palpable defect. This was substantiated arthroscopically in eight of eleven patients. One had only a torn meniscus; another had a partial tear of the anterior cruciate ligament that was not identified clinically. A third patient had degenerative arthritis in the medial compartment, which produced acute pain in the area of the tibial collateral ligament.

Torn anterior cruciate ligaments were commonly accompanied by a torn meniscus, usually laterally. The value of arthroscopy in acute ligamentous injury is identification of those patients for whom surgical intervention is indicated. It was learned from posterior puncture that acute anterior cruciate ligament injury is not isolated; it is always accompanied by hemorrhagic changes in either the posteromedial or posterolateral capsule and either a torn meniscus or a loose body.

In all 49 patients (16%) had a postarthroscopic diagnosis of torn anterior cruciate ligament. Of these patients, 24 were thought to have meniscal abnormalities as the primary diagnosis; patellar disease was suspected in one; and 34 had been classified as having an extrasynovial or ligamentous lesion.

Seven patients had a tear or attenuation in the anterior cruciate ligament; all had hemorrhage.

Most patients with a torn anterior cruciate ligament had an associated abnormality; the most common being a meniscal tear in 37% and degenerative arthritis in 22%.

Of continued concern were eight patients who had had a previous meniscectomy through a short anterior incision in the presence of a torn anterior cruciate ligament. They remained symptomatic, with either a large meniscus that was catching and popping in the posterior compartment or degenerative arthritis with loose bodies. It was common to find a subtotal meniscectomy with an existing old tear of the posterior horn behind the line of meniscal resection.

Two patients had a torn anterior cruciate ligament accompanying an acute dislocation of the patella. These were not recognizable clinically because the patients' pain limited the physical examination.

Synovial disease. In a number of patients only primary synovial disease was suspected. However, some had acute inflammatory degenerative arthritis with loose bodies causing a synovial reaction, and others had intermittent joint pain and swelling not established by arthroscopic examination. Other abnormalities observed included gout, pseudogout, pigmented villa nodular synovitis, and osteochondromatosis. Osteochondromatosis was managed in three patients without synovectomy but by vacuuming loose bodies from the joint; they have remained aysmptomatic for over a year.

Arthroscopy is of benefit in synovial diseases for establishing the conditions morphologically and providing access for biopsy. Appropriate medical and surgical recommendations can then be made.

Series III

Patients in Series III had *not* had recent arthroscopy; however, on the basis of history, physical examination, and x-ray findings, surgical exploration of the knee was warranted. All patients were given general anesthetic, and arthroscopy was carried out immediately prior to arthrotomy.

All patients in Series III were from my private practice. Only a few had medicolegal or Workmen's Compensation claims. Of the 150 patients, 122 were male and 28 were female. Their median age was 28 years.

Twelve patients had bilateral conditions, either a meniscal abnormality in the opposite compartment or bilateral patellar conditions; a few patients had bilateral degenerative disease or osteochondritis dissecans.

The preoperative diagnosis was substantiated in 54% of the patients, and an additional significant abnormality was identified in 22%. Clinical diagnosis was incorrect in 20%, and in 4% no abnormality was found within the joint, despite anterior, posteromedial, and posterolateral inspection and auxillary suprapatellar puncture.

Meniscal disease. Meniscal abnormalities most often misdiagnosed were an accompanying tear or an isolated tear of the meniscus in an opposite compartment. Some patients had loose bodies that mimicked a torn meniscus, and in three instances an acute dislocation of the patella with marked knee swelling was mistaken for an acute meniscal lesion.

Patellar conditions. In the patellar group, it was more common that a presumptive diagnosis was substantiated arthroscopically and surgically. In those patients with dislocations of the patella, one had a tear of the posterolateral meniscus identified only through that arthroscopic approach, and two patients had additional loose bodies. One patient was thought to have a ruptured patellar tendon, because of inability to extend the knee. The tendon was normal, but there was acute synovitis of the joint of a rheumatologic type.

Condylar disease. Suspected condylar disease was usually substantiated by arthroscopy. A few patients in this group had additional loose bodies.

Fifteen patients were treated arthroscopically, usually for loose bodies that mimicked some other condition. The loose bodies were removed either by vacuuming or with the Jaws modified pituitary ronjeur under arthroscopic control.

Extrasynovial lesions. Patients thought to have extrasynovial lesions, torn ligaments, or old instability of the joint most commonly had an unsuspected meniscal tear. In a few patients with massive hemarthrosis with mild instability, torn cruciate ligaments were clinically diagnosed on the basis of a twisting injury, an acute pop in the knee, and massive hemarthrosis. Arthroscopic inspection showed that these patients had a torn meniscus.

Patients with ligament injuries often have an additional torn meniscus. An isolated meniscal tear or an acute dislocation can mimic a ligament injury.

Synovial disease. Prior to synovectomy in one patient with rheumatoid changes in the knee, arthroscopy was carried out to substantiate synovitis and to rule out joint thickening as the basis of capsular thickening.

MANAGEMENT

In 23% of patients who had arthroscopy with general anesthetic, anterior inspection showed normal findings, yet posterior puncture showed a lesion. Twelve patients had an abnormality seen in the medial meniscus only from the posterior puncture. In five patients posterolateral inspection demonstrated a torn meniscus. In five patients no abnormality was seen in either the anteromedial or anterolateral compartment, yet they had a tear in both the posteromedial and posterolateral menisci not seen from the front.

It should be noted that loose bodies in either the posterior or posterolateral compartments were of significant size or quantity. Multiple small loose bodies were suctioned out through a cannula. The larger ones were removed with a Jaws modified pituitary ronjeur. Such removal prevents slowing of the rehabilitative process.

Arthroscopic observations of meniscal degeneration have improved understanding of meniscal conditions. The recognition that fringe tears can mimic a complete tear explains the negative findings of exploratory surgery in the past. Fringe tears can produce a positive McMurray sign, yet when the knee is opened, cleaned, and dried, the lesion is not visible to the naked eye. In the past, unnecessary meniscectomies have been performed to alleviate symptoms. However, the fringe tear will cleanse itself and the signs and symptoms will disappear (see Chapter 8).

Surgery was contemplated for 158 knees examined. Bilateral conditions, usually patellar subluxation requiring only lateral capsular release, were eliminated from the series. Surgery as proposed was carried out in 62% of patients. Arthroscopy immediately preceding surgery altered the exposure or design in 20%. Many of these patients had a tear of the opposite meniscus, some with no abnormality in the side of the referred pain, in addition to the lesion clinically anticipated. More important, 10% of the patients were treated arthroscopically, usually by removal of loose bodies not requiring surgical intervention. Heretofore these patients would have undergone arthrotomy.

Eight percent of the patients did not require surgery or arthroscopic management. It is significant that in 4% of patients, or six of those whom we thought had a torn medial meniscus, no diagnosis was substantiated. On three occasions a torn medial meniscus and was diagnosed clinically, but arthroscopy prior to arthrotomy established a dislocation of the patella. On four occasions a torn lateral meniscus was misdiagnosed as a torn medial meniscus. One patient had a torn lateral meniscus and an additional medial meniscal tear that required surgery.

Twenty-one patients who had ligamentous instability were given a general anesthetic before an anticipated arthrotomy. Eight of those 21 patients had a medial compartment instability with an unsuspected torn lateral meniscus, most commonly identified only by the posterolateral puncture. Again arthroscopy altered the surgical design. The significance is not so much that there was a clinical diagnostic error in 18% of patients, but rather that 18% of the patients did not undergo unnecessary arthrotomy, which would not have been beneficial.

It should be noted that 15 patients who were treated arthroscopically all had loose bodies, many in the posterior compartment. In the extrasynovial conditions with ligamentous injuries, eight of the 30 patients, or almost one third, had accompanying torn lateral menisci, many observed only by the posterolateral puncture.

The other large group for which surgery was altered had meniscal lesions with an additional anterior cruciate ligament tear catching in the lateral joint line and requiring surgical resection. Two patients had additional loose bodies. Three patients had a surprising amount of articular cartilage injury necessitating chondroplasty, which was not suggested on preoperative x-ray films. Six patients had an additional tear of the lateral meniscus; clinically they had medial meniscal symptoms only. One patient thought to have a lateral meniscal tear in fact had a medial meniscal abnormality.

VALUE OF ARTHROSCOPY

Arthroscopy has had, and continues to have a major impact on my clinical practice. This simple, efficient, practical diagnostic method has enhanced clinical skills and improved patient care. Arthroscopy has provided information that both dictated and contraindicated surgical intervention. No unnecessary incisions have been made. Loose bodies have been removed arthroscopically, thus avoiding arthrotomy. Patients have enjoyed a smoother rehabilitative process. At the same time, general understanding of meniscal degeneration, articular cartilage healing, and synovial morphologic patterns has increased. I would expect that others, regardless of clinical proficiency, would find similar benefits from inclusion of arthroscopy in their practice routine.

LEARNING ARTHROSCOPY

The following is offered as a method of becoming proficient in arthroscopy.

Short of individual instruction, which is difficult in arthroscopy, Instructional courses, reading materials, and audiovisual programs can be helpful. Nothing supersedes personal experience. The use of clinical models have limited value. The neophyte arthroscopist should obtain an above-the-knee amputation specimen and freeze it until a time when he is free to explore the joint. Because a cadaver is not supple and does not maintain distention well, arthroscopic viewing is difficult. A constricting tie around the thigh above the suprapatellar pouch will prevent leakage of saline. The amputation specimen femur may be clamped in a vise and draped as for surgery. The complete surgical setup, including presence of the assistant, will better prepare the potential arthroscopist for the procedure. After extensive viewing, the joint may be opened for the gross correlation of findings.

The first clinical arthroscopies should be performed on patients under general anesthesia for whom the surgeon anticipates arthrotomy. The arthroscopy should

74

be limited to 15 minutes, whether any viewing is accomplished or not. Prolonged viewing will bore the anesthesiologist and enrage the surgeons who are planning to follow you in the operating room suite. Both arthroscopy and the arthroscopist will acquire a bad reputation because of the inconvenience produced. With experience, the neophyte arthroscopist will become skilled enough to perform the complete arthroscopy in the allotted time. If no diagnosis is arrived at arthroscopically, one should proceed on the basis of clinical judgment. As the surgeon becomes more confident in his abilities, arthroscopy will influence decisions and even contradict preoperative clinical impressions. The contribution of arthroscopy to care of patients will be appreciated.

After technical confidence has been achieved, arthroscopy may be performed with the patient under local anesthesia. It is best to select confident and relaxed patient. The techniques are the same. The posteromedial approach will be easier to master than the posterolateral routine. With perserverance, most orthopedists will become competent in arthroscopy.

Appendix

TABLE 1. Series I: Prearthroscopic diagnosis

	Patients	Knees
Meniscal disease		
Torn medial meniscus	199	209
Torn lateral meniscus	29	29
Retained posterior horn	28	29
Miscellaneous evaluations	9	9
	265	276
Patellar disease		
Chondromalacia	35	37
Dislocation	7	7
Subluxation	7	9
Fracture	5	5
Parapatellar synovitis	2	2
Patellar prosthesis	1	1
Patella baja	1	1
	58	62
Condylar disease		
Degenerative articular cartilage	18	20
Osteochondritis dissecans	10	11
Loose bodies	5	5
	33	36
Extrasynovial disease		
Torn anterior cruciate ligament	17	18
Torn tibial collateral ligament	11	11
Baker's cyst	2	2
Ganglion cyst	1	1
	31	32
Synovial disease		
Synovitis	11	11
Foreign body	2	2
	13	13
	400	419

TABLE 2. Series I: Comparison of pre- and postarthroscopic diagnoses

	Postarthroscopic diagnosis			
	Correct		Incorrect	
Prearthroscopic diagnosis	Same (%)	Additional diagnosis (%)	Different diagnosis (%)	No diagnosis (%)
Meniscal disease				
Torn medial meniscus	24	12	40	24
Torn lateral meniscus	32	7	41	20
Retained posterior horn	62	32	6	
Miscellaneous evaluations				
Patellar disease				
Chondromalacia	56	30	14	
Dislocation		100		
Subluxation	50	50		
Fracture	60		40	
Parapatellar synovitis				
Patellar prosthesis				
Patella baja				
Condylar disease				
Degenerative articular cartilage	35	65		
Osteochondritis dissecans	100	100		
Loose bodies		100		
Extrasynovial disease				
Torn anterior cruciate ligament	36	45	19	
Torn tibial collateral ligament	61	39		
Baker's cyst				
Ganglion cyst				
Synovial disease				
Synovitis	100			
Foreign body	100			

TABLE 3. Series I: Prearthroscopic management

	Surgery	Arthroscopic management	Conservative treatment	Diagnosis only
Meniscal disease				
Torn medial meniscus	78	7	124	
Torn lateral meniscus	11		18	
Retained posterior horn	17	2	10	
Miscellaneous evaluations				9
Patellar disease				
Chondromalacia	2	3	32	
Dislocation	7			
Subluxation	6		3	
Fracture			5	
Parapatellar synovitis				2
Patellar prosthesis	1			
Patella baja	1			
Condylar disease				
Degenerative articular cartilage	4	0	16	
Osteochondritis dissecans	1	0	10	
Loose bodies	1	1	3	
Extrasynovial disease				
Torn anterior cruciate ligament	6	1	11	
Torn tibial collateral ligament	4		7	
Baker's cyst	2			
Ganglion cyst	1			
Synovial disease				
Synovitis				11
Foreign body	1		1	
	143 (34%)	14 (3%)	240 (57%)	22 (5%)

TABLE 4. Series I: Resultant management

	Surgery (%)	Arthroscopic management	Conservative treatment	Diagnosis only
All cases	34	3	57	5
Meniscal disease	38	3	56	3
Patellar disease	28	4	66	3
Condylar disease	17	3	80	
Extrasynovial disease	41	3	56	
Synovial disease	9	9		82

TABLE 5. Series II: Prearthroscopic diagnosis

	Knees
Meniscal disease	
Torn medical meniscus	115
Torn lateral meniscus	45
Retained posterior horn	21
Contusions	3
Miscellaneous evaluations	20
Patellar disease	
Chondromalacia	27
Dislocation	14
Subluxation	21
Contusion	4
Osteochondritis dissecans	2
Bipartite patella	1
Condylar disease	5
Degenerative articular cartilage	24
Osteochondritis dissecans	4
Loose bodies	10
Fracture	1
Extrasynovial disease	
Torn tibial collateral ligament	11
Torn anterior cruciate ligament	26
Torn fibular collateral ligament	1
Torn posterior cruciate ligament	1
Rotary instability	9
Synovial disease	
Synovitis	19
	384

TABLE 6. Series II: Comparison of pre- and postarthroscopic diagnoses

| | Postarthroscopic diagnosis | | | |
| | Correct | | Incorrect | |
Prearthroscopic diagnosis	Same (%)	Additional diagnosis (%)	Different diagnosis (%)	No diagnosis (%)
Meniscal disease				
Torn medial meniscus	31	16	23	30
Torn lateral meniscus	35	7	40	18
Retained posterior horn	28	62	10	
Miscellaneous evaluations				
Patellar disease				
Chondromalacia	55	20	5	20
Dislocation	14	85		
Subluxation	33	33	16	17
Contusion				
Osteochondritis dissecans				
Bipartite patella				
Condylar disease				
Degenerative articular cartilage	66	24	10	
Osteochondritis dissecans	100			
Loose bodies	90	10		
Fracture				
Extrasynovial disease				
Torn tibial collateral ligament	73	18	9	
Torn anterior cruciate ligament	19	70	11	
Torn fibular collateral ligament				
Torn posterior cruciate ligament				
Rotary instability				
Synovial disease				
Synovitis	50	50		

TABLE 7. Series III: Comparison of pre- and postarthroscopic diagnosis

Prearthroscopic diagnosis	Postarthroscopic diagnosis			
	Correct		Incorrect	
	Same	Additional diagnosis	Different diagnosis	No diagnosis
Meniscal disease				
Torn medial meniscus	35	13	20	6
Torn lateral meniscus	5	8	4	
Retained posterior horn		3		
Patellar disease				
Chondromalacia	1			
Dislocation	8	3		
Subluxation	7			
Ruptured tendon			1	
Patellectomy	1			
Condylar disease				
Degenerative articular cartilage	7	2		
Degenerative meniscal tear		1		
Osteochondritis dissecans	3			
Loose bodies	4			
Extrasynovial disease				
Torn anterior cruciate ligament	4	3	6	
Torn tibial collateral ligament	2	1	2	
Old instability	3	2		
Cyst	3			
Ankylosis	1			
Osgood-Schlatter disease	1			
Synovial disease				
Synovitis	1			
	87 (54%)	36 (22%)	33 (20%)	6 (4%)

TABLE 8. Management of 158 knees for which surgery was contemplated

	Surgery as proposed	Surgery altered	Arthroscopically managed	Surgery not indicated
Meniscal disease	59	23	3	8
Patellar disease	18		2	1
Condylar disease	8		7	1
Extrasynovial disease	13	8	2	3
Synovial disease	1			
	62%	20%	10%	8%

Of 82% undergoing surgery, 62% had surgery as proposed; for 20% there was change in surgical design. Ten percent were arthroscopically managed. In 8%, neither surgery nor arthroscopy was required.

TABLE 9. Altered surgery

	Meniscal disease	Extrasynovial disease
Medial meniscus tear plus anterior cruciate tear	4	
Medial meniscus tear plus loose bodies	2	
Medial meniscus tear plus severe degenerative arthritis	3	
Medial meniscus tear plus torn lateral meniscus	6	
No medial meniscus tear but dislocation of patella	3	
No medial meniscus tear but tear of lateral meniscus	4	
Lateral meniscus tear plus medial meniscus tear	1	
Torn ligament plus unsuspected torn lateral meniscus		8

TABLE 10. Value of posterior punctures

	Number of knees	Postero-medial	Postero-lateral	Both	Loose bodies
Meniscal disease	18 of 88	9	2	2	5
Patellar disease	3 of 16				3
Condylar disease	4 of 15				4
Extrasynovial disease	11 of 30	3	3	3	2
Synovial disease	0 of 1				
	36 of 150	12	5	5	14
	23%				

Chapter 6

Documentation

Dictated narrative
Chart documentation
Still photography
    Camera adapters
    Film
Movie photography
Television

Immediate documentation following arthroscopy is essential. Experience has shown that time lapse between end of the procedure and documentation of findings (i.e., for performance of another arthroscopic examination) results in greatly diminished recall. Therefore, a dictated narrative should be made immediately following the procedure—before phone calls, patient discharge, or extraneous conversation.

DICTATED NARRATIVE

The narrative entered on the outpatient report should include a brief history and results of physical examination of the patient (box, p. 83). Prearthroscopic diagnosis and postarthroscopic findings are documented. The procedure is always recorded in a routine manner, regardless of how it was technically accomplished.

Findings in the patella and suprapatellar pouch are recorded first, because this area is usually examined first. However, in patients with tight, fat, or scarred knees, complete inspection under the patella is not possible from the initial anteromedial puncture, and the area must be inspected later in the procedure by auxillary suprapatellar puncture. Findings are still recorded first.

The next paragraph describes the anterolateral compartment, its meniscal substance, and its articular surface in the tangential view.

Findings in the intercondylar notch are described next in a separate paragraph, including status of the fat pad, size, fibrosis, and ecchymosis, as well as inspection of the anterior cruciate ligament and the presence of loose bodies.

Documentation of the anteromedial compartment includes findings on the articular surface and in the meniscal substance, extent of examination, any limitations due to mechanical tightness inherent in the knee, and technical problems.

Findings in the posteromedial compartment include those of the articular surface and the meniscus, as well as the presence of loose bodies or synovitis and the status of the posterior cruciate ligament. This compartment is not inspected if anteromedial findings indicate that surgical exploration is warranted.

Recorded findings in the posterolateral compartment include the status of the meniscus and articular surface of the posterior femoral condyle. Occasionally it is

Example of dictated narrative

The patient is a 28-year-old white man who has had previous medial and lateral meniscectomies, with attenuation of the anterior cruciate ligament. He has catching and pain on the outer aspect of the right knee in spite of lateral meniscectomy. Arthrography does not show any specific abnormality at this time.

Physical examination shows a stable patella and a relatively stable knee, with only minimal evidence of anterior cruciate laxity. There is some crepitus over the lateral joint line in the lateral femoral condyle, but no acute tenderness, no heat, no effusion.

Clinical diagnosis. Status postoperative medial and lateral meniscectomies, right knee: partial tear in anterior cruciate ligament.

Preoperative diagnosis. Status postoperative medial and lateral meniscectomies: partial tear in anterior cruciate ligament.

Postoperative diagnosis.
1. Posterior horn in lateral meniscus
2. Degenerative arthritis, moderately severe, in lateral femoral condyle
3. Status postoperative medial meniscectomy
4. Attenuated anterior cruciate ligament

Procedure. The patient was placed on a table. A tourniquet was placed high on the right thigh. The entire right knee was prepared with Betadine and sterile draped so as to expose the area.

Plain lidocaine 1% was injected into the infrapatellar fat pad and the infrapatellar branch of the saphenous nerve. A sharp and then a blunt trocar were placed in the joint, and the joint was distended with saline.

The undersurface of the patella was seen and found to be smooth. There is mild synovitis of the joint. Minimal stardusting was vacuumed out of the joint.

The lateral compartment shows diffuse degenerative articular changes, chunky and fibrillar in nature.

The lateral meniscus shows rather prominent size near the area of the posterior horn and some tibial condylar fibrillation.

The intercondylar notch shows an attenuated anterior cruciate ligament.

The medial compartment shows a small regenerated meniscus and no articular injury.

A separate posteromedial puncture shows only a minimal remnant of the posterior meniscus, with no separation.

A separate posterolateral puncture shows a rather large posterior lateral meniscus. The meniscus was palpated and popped back and forth. The patient feels that this duplicates his symptoms of instability in the lateral joint line.

The fluid and equipment were removed. A sterile dressing was applied, and the patient was taken to the recovery room in good condition.

Recommendations. I would recommend arthrotomy through a transverse skin incision after the fashion of Bruser, with the patient in a cross-legged position. The posterior horn of the lateral meniscus should be removed. Some shaving of the lateral femoral condyle might be in order. The patient should be told that the prognosis is not good because of the presence of degenerative lateral compartment disease.

possible to describe the popliteus tendon and its sheath, as well as the presence of loose bodies.

Any technical problems are documented, as is the completeness of the examination. Occasionally there are limitations to areas inspected, which should be noted as due to technical inability, scar tissue, obesity, or lack of cooperation of the patient.

The last paragraph includes recommendations, whether the patient was referred only for consultation or is going to be treated directly.

CHART DOCUMENTATION

When the patient record is dictated, the postarthroscopic diagnosis and date are written on the patient's office chart, in case the dictation is lost.

Diagrams, charts, and drawings can be helpful, especially early in arthroscopic experience; familiarity with arthroscopic descriptions diminishes the usefulness of diagrams. The diagram shown in Fig. 6-1 serves for both right and left knees. A more definitive illustration of findings can be added, including those from the posteromedial and posterolateral compartments.

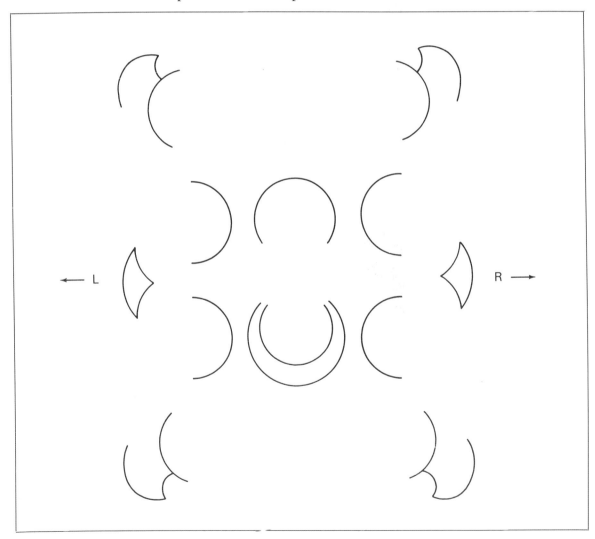

FIG. 6-1. This diagram serves as basis for further descriptive drawings.

STILL PHOTOGRAPHY

There is a universal desire by those embarking on arthroscopy to produce photographic documentation. Even a hazy, poorly illuminated, artistically and photographically uninteresting slide will excite the novice arthroscopist. A slide of a lesion may be of interest to the arthroscopist and the patient, but with the passage of time it will bring only a ho-hum reaction from even the arthroscopist.

Slide photography has some limitations because of the number of frames on any given roll of film. By the time the film has been developed, much of the arthroscopy has been forgotten. Unless one is very compulsive about record keeping (i.e., identifying film as to the exact patient, compartments, and findings), there frequently will be many slides of little recognizable value. Also, with hundreds of slides, many will be duplications. Slide photography is not a practical recording method except for rare cases, medicolegal claims, or for establishing a slide file for teaching purposes.

Photography is a function of light that produces an image on photographic film. In arthroscopy, the variables are the amount of light that can be thrown on an object and the amount of light that can come back through the lens of the endoscope. It is axiomatic that the smaller the diameter of the endoscope, the smaller the amount of light that can be thrown on the object. The smaller the diameter of the arthroscopic lens, the smaller the amount of light that can be transmitted to the film. Therefore, the smaller endoscopes have less photographic capacity. The quality varies with the amount of light thrown on the subject. An excellent photograph is less likely with the 1.7-mm diameter Needlescope than with an endoscope of 5- to 6.5-mm diameter.

Other variables include the transmission of light along fiberglass bundles. If there is breakage of the fiber bundles, which occurs over a period of time, or corrosion over the end of the bundles, there will be diminution of light transmission (see Chapter 2).

Most available illuminators provide ample light for viewing with any endoscope. The quality of the illuminator is more critical with the smaller diameter endoscopes and fiberoptic bundle mass. The more powerful output will throw more light on an object; hence, viewing will be clearer. It is my opinion that the serious arthroscopist will require a Dyonics Model 500 illuminator or a Storz xenon light source for optimal viewing and photography.

It should be noted that light bulbs lose power with time. Before they burn or wear out, light can be diminished to a rather significant degree, at least for photographic or television documentation. Thus, for excellent photographic work, frequent bulb changes are indicated. The Sylvania Colorarc 300/16 lamp produces more light than does the General Electric Marc 300/16 projection lamp, as documented photographically.

Camera adapters

I first utilized a single-lens reflex camera with a universal lens attachment, manufactured by the Dyonics Corporation. A high-density plastic screw secures the ocular lens very snugly, which permits freedom of motion for photographic purposes (Fig. 6-2). I prefer the half-frame camera to the full-frame, because the image has less black border around it and projects a cleaner image on the photographic screen. I have continued to use this particular equipment because it does not have a long lens that further increases the lever arm on the equipment. Recent modifications are easily attached and securely hold the camera to the eyepiece. It will fit all endoscope ocular lenses. The "thumb-pinch" type of attachment does not provide a firm attachment to the ocular lens of the arthroscope.

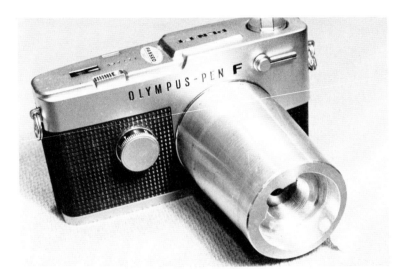

FIG. 6-2. Universal lens attachment permits freedom of motion for photographic purposes.

Film

I originally used Kodak Ektachrome ASA-64 film, the Dyonics Model 400 illuminator, and shutter speeds in the range of 1/8 to 1/30 second. When the slides were edited correctly and enough of the bright femoral condyle and meniscus was included, the image could be documented. Photography improved with adoption of a light source in the 550-K range, the Dyonics Model 500 Fiberoptic Illuminator (see Fig. 2-5), which provided increased photographic capacity even in dimly lit areas on slides. I switched to the high-speed Ektachrome ASA-160 film, which can be pushed to an ASA of 1,000 during processing (Fig. 6-3, A), thus improving documentation of darkened recesses of the knee. The Dyonics Model III Needlescope produces a good photograph with a Storz flash generator and Kodachrome ASA-64 film. This model has a wide angle of view, compared with that of the Needlescope Model II (Fig. 6-3, B). With the small-diameter arthroscopes, consistently good black-and-white reprints can be produced with Kodak 2475 recording film exposed at 1/15 second and with standard processing. This is even possible using the 2.2-mm Needlescope and the regular Dyonics illuminator. Although black-and-white photographs made with regular stock film can be used, there is some graininess and they do not have the sharpness of color prints.

Consistently good films can be made with either the Dyonics rod-lens scope or the Storz-Hopkins rod-lens system. The Dyonics rod-lens system (Fig. 6-3, *C*) provides a wide angle of view of the entire meniscus and the femoral condyle. Methylene blue was placed in the joint for contrast. The Storz flash generator and Ektachrome ASA-64 film were used. The Storz 4-mm endoscope (Fig. 6-3, *D*) also allows a wide angle of view. The light source used was the Storz flash generator; the film was Kodachrome ASA-64. A yellowish photograph is typical because of the light balance with this endoscope and film and does not represent pathologic abnormality. For photographic purposes, the rod lens has less stigmatism and color aberration. This is not necessarily apparent to the eye, but can be seen by comparison of photographs.

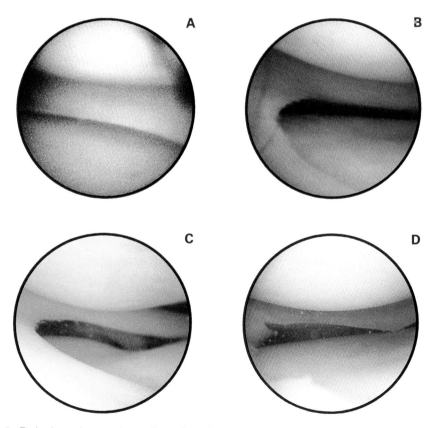

FIG. 6-3. Relative size and quality of endoscopic pictures taken with various endoscopes. **A,** Original Needlescope with available light. **B,** Model III Needlescope with flash generator. **C,** Dyonics rod lens with flash generator. Methylene blue is utilized as contrast medium. **D,** Endoscopic view taken with Storz rod-lens scope with flash generator.

The best photographic slide documents that I have seen have been made with the Storz flash generator, which produces abundant light for excellent photography and has an advantage in that the flash unit is attached to the endoscope. Flash units that have their origin within the light box lose a considerable amount of potential light. A percentage of the effective light is lost for every foot it travels down a fiberoptic cable. Most light cables are 6 feet long. Therefore, if the flash unit is within the box, 48% of the potential light is lost. In addition, 30% of the light is lost at each interphase. These high light losses are reduced by the Storz flash generator because the source is attached directly to the endoscope (Fig. 6-4).

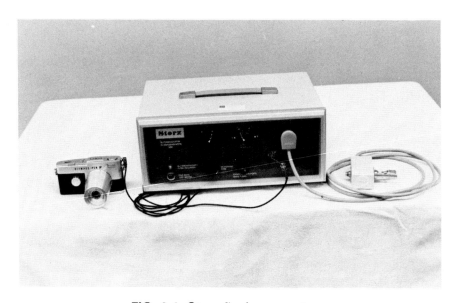

FIG. 6-4. Storz flash generator.

MOVIE PHOTOGRAPHY

Movie photography has a definite advantage in that the entire arthroscopic examination is duplicated on film (Fig. 6-5).

Composition not possible with still photography is most effective, and observation of the flow of fluid and the motion of the intra-articular tissues (i.e., synovium, menisci, or loose bodies) is valuable. This method of documentation is somewhat impractical, however, because of the high cost of the film and the expense and weight of the equipment.

Good photography was achieved with the 8-mm Beaulieu direct-viewing, motor-driven, Super 8 camera with Ektachrome-7241 high-speed single-perforated film. However, because this film did not lock solidly during exposure, I switched to a 16-mm Beaulieu camera with 7241 double-perforated film (Fig. 6-6). It was necessary to use the Dyonics Model 500 Fiberoptic 500-K illuminator in order to achieve enough light. With an additional light source (i.e., a light wand), it is possible to photograph with the 1.7-mm scope. Adequate photography can be accomplished using the 2.2-mm diameter scope with the light provided within its cannula. Because areas in the distant range are rather dark, a circumferential halo

FIG. 6-5. Cinephotography provides best method of documenting endoscopic views.

A Lateral femoral condyle is superior, and meniscus with irregularity along its inner border is to left.
B Deeper, posterior horn of meniscus comes into view.
C Needlescope, 2.2-mm diameter, under meniscus.
D Further penetration of endoscope shows horizontal cleft tear in undersurface of meniscus.
E Retraction of endoscope shows elevated inner border of meniscus. Tear was identified only by proceeding under meniscus with small-diameter endoscope. Dynamics of pistoning are well illustrated.

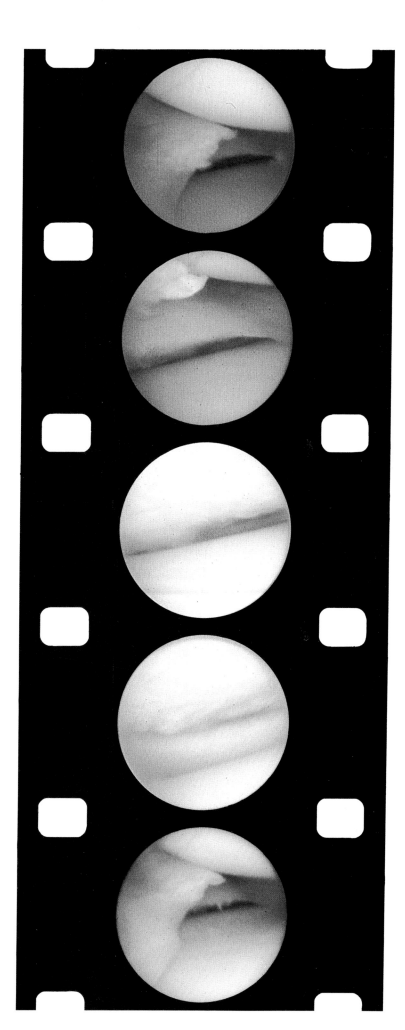

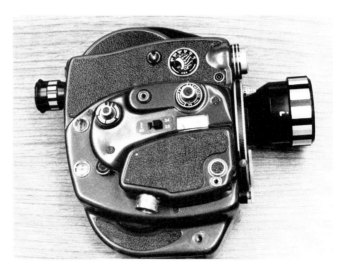

FIG. 6-6. Beaulieu 16-mm movie camera with Dyonics lens mount.

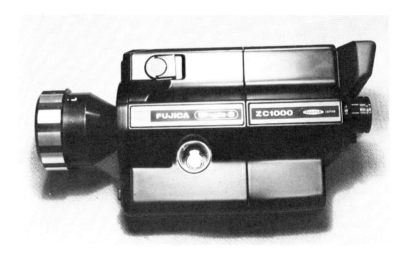

FIG. 6-7. Fuji XL 1000 Single Eight movie camera is cassette loaded.

light was devised, which increases the light by 16 times, producing an excellent image.

Cinephotography with the Storz 3.5- and 5-mm endoscopes produces sharp, clear, well-illuminated photographs. We have utilized the Dyonics 76 rod lens system with similar photography capacity.

Although the Dyonics rod-lens system has a slightly narrower field of view, it focuses closer to the object than does the Storz 5-mm endoscope. The choice between them is a matter of the user's preference.

More recently we have utilized the Fuji XL-1000 camera body with a Dyonics lens attachment and a C-mount connector, with Fuji ASA-200 film (Fig. 6-7). This system is lightweight, battery-driven, and easily loaded with a single 8 cassette. The photographic image has excellent illumination but appears somewhat grainy. Fugi ASA-400 film should be available in the near future. Because films come in single rolls of 50 feet, they are excellent for record keeping. They are viewed on

Super 8 viewing devices or projector equipment, which many arthroscopists already have for home movie systems.

TELEVISION

With the advent of modern technology in videotape equipment, it is possible to document endoscopy with television cassettes.[1] Because there is no wait for film to be developed, what was observed through the endoscope can be reviewed immediately. Adequacy of the arthroscopic examination can be confirmed, or if a part of it was not satisfactory, it can be repeated right away. Some findings can be observed on the television screen that are not seen by direct vision.

Television cassette recording was of further advantage in consultation work. The patient can deliver the cassette with the audiovisual record of the endoscopy to the referring physician, eliminating any delay in the transmission of written records and visual documentation. The referring physician can mail the cassette back for reuse. Videotape also has proved to be of value in documenting and storing good cases for teaching purposes. The use of the counter on the recording device isolates the area of any given arthroscopy.

The Medic III television system consists of a free-standing, movable cabinet with locking doors in both front and rear. The monitor mount is capable of 350° rotation without destroying or entangling the cables. It has an adequate storage area below for tapes and accessories. Sliding shelves provide easy access to both the camera and the videotape recording equipment. A formica surface ensures the continued handsome appearance of the cabinet (Fig. 6-8).

The system has three basic pieces of equipment: color camera, a cassette videotape recorder, and a color monitor.

The camera is a single-tube color camera with a remote-control unit and 15 feet of interconnecting cable. The camera head weighs less than 4 pounds. It is supplied with a 25-mm lens with a 16-mm C-mount for clinical documentation

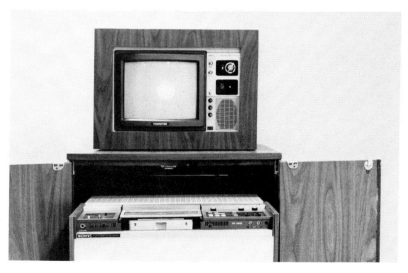

FIG. 6-8. Videotape has proved to be excellent means of recording endoscopic abnormalities. (Equipment assembled by R. P. Hermes Co., Detroit.)

other than arthroscopy. There are 250 television lines and horizontal resolution, as well as a built-in color-bar generator for precision setup.

The color-videotape recorder uses 3/4-inch cassettes. It has a positive freeze-frame control. A built-in headphone jack provides for personal or private review of the material, as well as for sound dubbing. There is a remote control unit with 15 feet of cable, so the circulating nurse can manage the system.

The color monitor, a 12-inch in-line Trinitron Plus picture tube, is capable of standard telecast and closed-circuit television signals. It has an automatic color switch and automatic fine tuning.

A suspension system for the camera is under design investigation and trial and when completed will facilitate the use of videotape equipment.

REFERENCE

1. McGinty, J. A.: Closed circuit television in arthroscopy, Int. Rev. Rheumatol., special edition devoted to arthroscopy, pp. 45-49, 1976.

Chapter 7

Arthroscopic anatomy

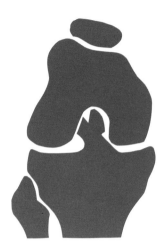

Normal arthroscopic anatomy
Anatomic compartments: technique and pathology
    Anterolateral compartment
    Intercondylar notch
    Anteromedial compartment
    Posteromedial compartment
    Posterolateral compartment

NORMAL ARTHROSCOPIC ANATOMY

A recognition of the normal anatomy and its variants is essential to any pathologic interpretation. The opportunity to perform arthroscopy on patients as young as 3 years of age and as old as 70 has allowed an understanding of the normal anatomy for any given age and an appreciation of normal degenerative changes. The following description and illustrations will help to establish a basis from which change can be recognized.

In the knee joint of a person under the age of 15 years, the meniscus is thin in the anteroposterior and vertical dimensions. There is a very sharp inner margin without degenerative changes. The meniscus lies flat and very close to the tibial condyle. Even when valgus strain is applied to the knee, the meniscus elevates only slightly off the condyle. There is a smooth transition from the meniscus to the synovium.

Views of the meniscus from the posteromedial and posterolateral compartments show a clean junction with the articular cartilage. There is no pile up of synovium at the posterior slope of the meniscus, and the contour is smooth, with no irregularities. The meniscus fits firmly against the condylar surfaces.

Articular cartilage in the preadolescent is absolutely smooth, usually white, and has no areas of roughening (Fig. 7-1, *A* and *B*).

The ligamentous tissue is easily identified. Frequently, a well-formed blood vessel is seen running the length of the synovium on the cruciate ligament (Fig. 7-1, *B*). With a drawer test it is easy to discern minimal normal laxity in that ligament. With anterior displacement of the tibia on the femur, there is minimal motion and rapid tightening of the anterior cruciate ligament. It also is apparent that there is a twisting and untwisting of the anterior cruciate fibers during tightening and relaxation, very much as if they were constructed like cable. Because there is generally no overlying fat, the cable appearance of the anterior cruciate ligament is seen beneath the synovium.

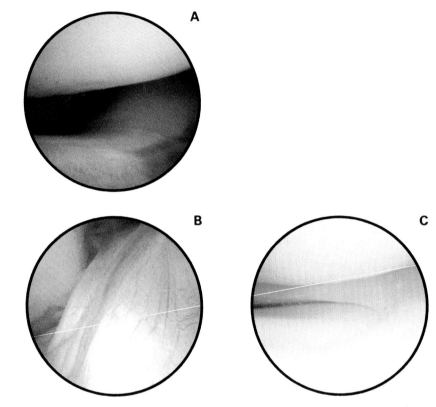

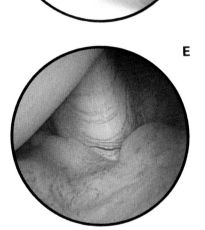

FIG. 7-1

A Suprapatellar pouch. Patella superior; intercondylar notch below. Notice normal vascularity of synovium.

B Intercondylar notch. Anterior cruciate ligament in midportion. Blood vessel on anterior cruciate ligament is normal.

C Medial compartment seen in its entirety with rod-lens endoscope. Femoral condyle superior. Methylene blue utilized for contrast.

D Meniscal-synovial reflection normal. Femoral condyle superior. Tibial collateral ligament prominent with valgus stress.

E Posteromedial compartment. Normal posterior cruciate ligament. Posterior femoral condyle to left.

The tibial collateral ligament has a prominence immediately subsynovial, adjacent to the meniscus and in the slot medial to the medial femoral condyle. It is possible with valgus strain on the knee to bring this ligament into relief to demonstrate its integrity (Fig. 7-1, *D*).

The posterior cruciate ligament can be seen easily in posteromedial inspection as it courses from the posterior aspect of the tibia up into the intercondylar notch (Fig. 7-1, *E*).

The popliteus tendon can be seen in three different areas. From an anteromedial approach, it is visible under the lateral meniscus, where it courses through the area devoid of coronary ligament (Fig. 7-2, *B*). Its attachment is seen from an anterolateral approach down the sulcus lateral to the femoral condyle (Fig. 7-2, *C*). The most complete inspection of the popliteus tendon is carried out from the posterolateral approach. It is often possible to pick up the course of that tendon and follow down its sheath as it courses posterior and inferior to the meniscus (Fig. 7-2, *D*). The tendon has a silvery appearance in a young person, and cross-hatching of collagen bundles is often apparent.

The synovium is flat, with only a rare villous formation. Normally, only a fine pattern of vascularity is observed (Fig. 7-2, *E*).

During adolescence the meniscus begins to degenerate. The first sign is translucency of its inner border; otherwise, there are no significant findings that could be considered normal. It should be noted that those individuals who are involved in vigorous athletic endeavors will have earlier degenerative meniscal changes, possibly including early fringe fragmentation. If there has been some significant injury, fragmentation of the meniscus or injury to the articular surfaces may result.

In teenaged girls the patellar surface is normally smooth, but there may be shaggy synovial fronds hanging about the patella. Often these become symptomatic if they are caught between the patella and the femoral condyle. Synovial fronds can become hemorrhagic, mimicking chondromalacia patellae. In many young girls, patellar pain and positive findings of patellar crepitus are not due to articular surface changes but to catching of the parapatellar synovium.

In the third decade of life, fringe degeneration of the meniscus including fringe tags is common. Normally, the brilliant white cartilage seen in the young knee starts to take on a yellow hue. The synovium is more villous and a bit more vascular.

Over the subsequent decades, it is common for degenerative changes of the meniscus to increase. The meniscus may develop yellow streaks. Thickened areas in the meniscus make its surfaces smooth and rounded. It increases in girth. Posteromedial and posterolateral punctures show the meniscus to have convoluted rather than smooth surfaces.

The articular surfaces lose their brilliance and sharp edges. The first sign of degenerative change is a smooth cobblestoning, which can advance to complete loss of articular surface and the uncovering of yellow bone (see Chapter 8). The normal degenerative process can include development of osteophytes. The synovium becomes considerably more villous and proliferative, especially in the posteromedial and posterolateral compartments. Projections are seen coming off the posteromedial and posterolateral synovial reflections of the meniscus.

FIG. 7-2

A Anterolateral compartment. Entire lateral meniscus, with femoral condyle superior. Methylene blue used in joint for contrast.

B By pistoning toward posterolateral corner of lateral compartment, popliteus tendon can be seen under meniscus. No coronary ligament in area, and popliteus tendon seen beyond notch in tibial surface.

C Anterolateral approach down sulcus, above popliteus tendon. Lateral femoral condyle is to right. Opening seen beyond is into posterolateral compartment. Popliteus tendon inferior, between 5 and 6 o'clock.

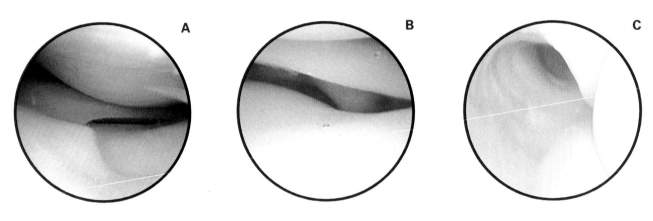

D Posterolateral approach. Normal femoral-condylar-meniscal junction. Meniscus has no tears. Normal synovial vascularity on posterior wall. No loose bodies.

E Posterolateral compartment. Popliteus tendon crossing obliquely, going down its sheath beneath and posterior to meniscus. Femoral condyle superior. Methylene blue utilized for contrast. It is possible to pass small-diameter endoscope down popliteus sheath to vacuum out loose bodies, if they exist.

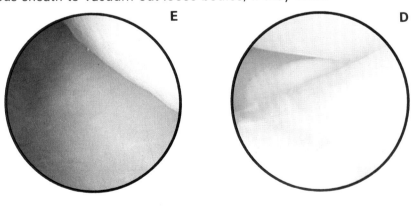

There is a time at which the normal degenerative changes in the knee take on clinical importance. Histologic sectioning of torn menisci, even in young people, indicates that there has been prior degenerative meniscal change. It is apparent that a virgin meniscus does not tear, except perhaps off of the synovial attachment, in a young person. Severe degenerative meniscal changes are usually accompanied with instability and mechanical malalignment (i.e., tibia vara).

With the instillation of saline, it is not uncommon for a localized area of synovial fluid to appear syrupy (as one might see if sugar were dropped into a glass of water). This is normal. Otherwise, there should be no particles, or stardusting (see Chapter 8), in the synovial fluid. It is not uncommon for the saline to be rapidly engulfed by the synovium, where it appears as glistening little silver balls inside the synovial villae.

ANATOMIC COMPARTMENTS: TECHNIQUE AND PATHOLOGY

The technique as outlined in Chapter 3 illustrates the mechanics of entering the individual anatomic compartments of the knee. The arthroscopic views of each compartment are unique. For instance, the medial meniscus in a normal knee lies closer to the tibial condyle, even with valgus stress, than would the lateral meniscus with varus stress. The lateral meniscus tends to ride up off of the tibia in a normal knee. Anatomic landmarks are seen in specific compartments. The posterior cruciate ligament is seen only from the posteromedial puncture; the origin of the popliteus tendon is seen from an anterolateral approach, and through a posterolateral approach it can be seen coursing back behind the meniscus; the anterior cruciate ligament is seen only from the intercondylar view.

Some pathologic abnormalities are unique to a particular anatomic compartment. Compression fracture or articular defect of an acute dislocation of the patella is seen in the medial view of the anterolateral compartment, at a site one meniscus breadth superior and lateral to the meniscal-synovial reflection. It has been noted that most loose bodies collect in the posterolateral compartment as a result of gravity, because when a person sits, the thigh is normally in slight external rotation.

Each of the following sections illustrates an anatomic compartment. Technique is demonstrated, and the role of each member of the arthroscopic team in achieving visualization of that compartment is outlined. The facing pages show normal anatomic structures visualized in the area, as well as illustrations of pathologic abnormalities that are unique to the respective compartment.

Anterolateral compartment

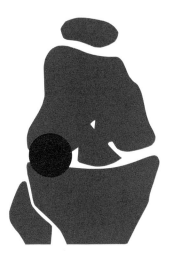

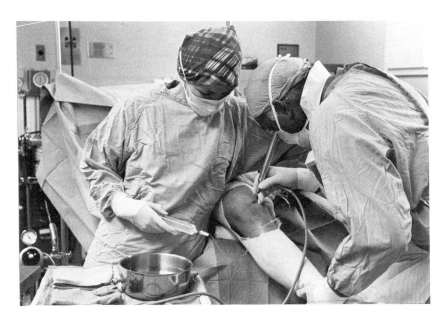

Patient The patient is supine on the table, with his legs hanging free over the end.

Assistant The assistant stands next to the patient's thigh and supports the inner distal femur with her hand.

Physician The physician stands. With his free hand, he applies varus stress to the knee, which when coupled with approximately 15° flexion of the knee usually opens the joint to maximum. In order to view a defect in the lateral femoral condyle, maximal distention, which pushes the synovium off the condyle, may be necessary. The physician may move to the lateral side of the patient's leg and apply varus strain with his hip and body. This frees both hands for inspection and cleansing.

FIG. 7-3

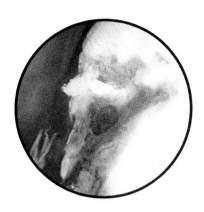

A Tangential view of lateral femoral condyle shows acute dislocation of patella. There also may be depression with roughening in subluxation of patella. Normal knee may have minimal depression without roughened articular surface. Loss of articular surface may accompany acute dislocations.

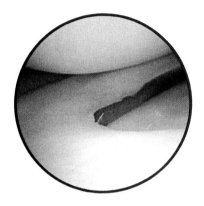

B Entire lateral meniscus. Femoral condyle is superior. Meniscus has sharp normal margins. Lateral meniscus elevates off tibial condyle with varus stress slightly more than medial meniscus would with valgus stress.

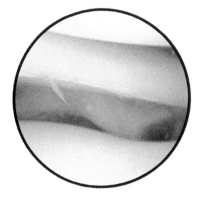

C Methylene blue in joint for contrast. View under lateral meniscus to area where popliteus tendon crosses posterolaterally. Area is devoid of coronary ligament. Tendon has lighter color of reflection than does meniscus, which assists in identification.

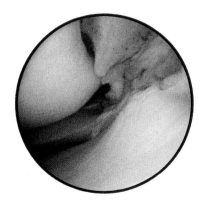

D Lateral compartment is first viewed adjacent to tibial spine. Landmark for orientation is junction between femoral condyle and tibial spine. Penetration brings posterior horn of lateral meniscus into view. Hemorrhage is seen in intercondylar notch.

Intercondylar notch

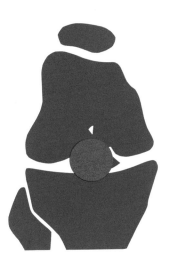

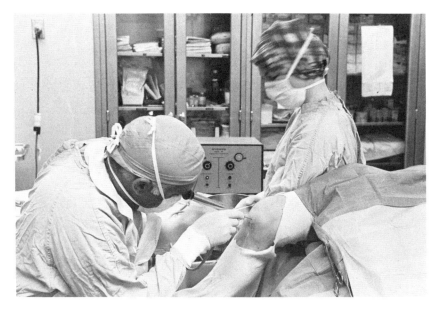

Patient The patient is supine, with his legs hanging free over the edge of the table.

Assistant The assistant stands next to the patient, stabilizing the distal thigh with her elbow or body.

Physician The physician sits with the patient's foot in his lap at between 45° and 90° flexion. It is possible to visualize the notch and perform a drawer test to document the integrity of the anterior cruciate ligament.

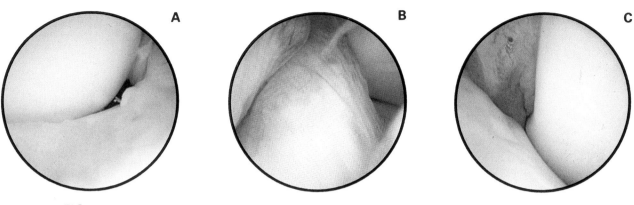

FIG. 7-4

A Junction of lateral femoral condyle and intercondylar notch is anatomic landmark.

B Anterior cruciate ligament with some increased vascularity but no tear. Medial approach reduces fat pad interference.

C Junction of medial femoral condyle and intercondylar notch. Notice synovial vascularity in foreground. Extreme anterior horn of meniscus seen in this area.

D Bucket-handle tear on lateral side of notch. Considerable synovitis and partial disruption of anterior cruciate ligament.

E Loose bodies in intercondylar notch can be removed with Jaws modified pituitary forceps while patient is under local anesthesia.

F Tear of anterior cruciate ligament, with massive disruption and hemorrhage. Direct preoperative evaluation of cruciate ligament provides evidence as to its integrity and repairability.

G Partial tear of anterior cruciate ligament caught in lateral joint line. Symptoms are similar to those of torn lateral meniscus. Treatment consists of resection of this portion of ligament.

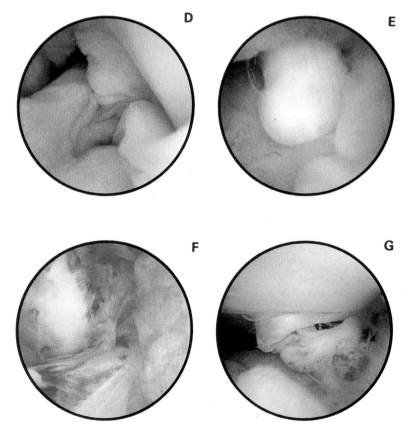

Anteromedial compartment

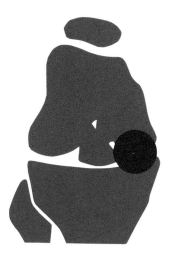

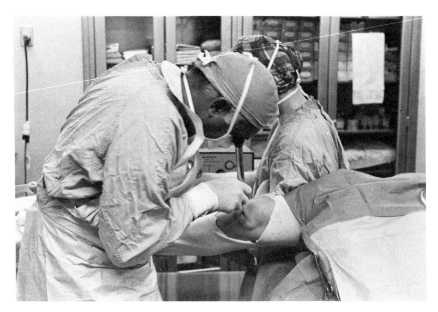

Patient   The patient is supine on the table, with his legs hanging free.

Assistant   The assistant stands to the patient's side and supports the distal femur with her elbow.

Physician   The physician stands and applies a valgus stress with his free hand. It may be necessary to flex and extend the patient's leg and rotate it internally and externally in order to complete the composite viewing of the medial compartment.

The original direction of entry is 30° laterally. However, redirection of the endoscope in a patient with scar or fat tissue may be necessary. Redirection should *not* be considered a lack of ability but a matter of appropriate technique. It is done by removing the endoscope and reinserting the blunt trocar. The cannula and trocar are retracted into the subcutaneous tissue. The capsule is repunctured toward the medial compartment.

FIG. 7-5

A Entire anteromedial compartment, with meniscus below femoral condyle.

B With valgus strain on knee, meniscus raises up in serpentine fashion. This amount of elevation normal in mobile knee joint. To move under meniscus, it is important that meniscus be elevated in this manner. Scope is then placed under an elevated area. Valgus stress is reduced for viewing under meniscus.

C With methylene blue in medial compartment, most extreme anterior portion of horn of meniscus seen at synovial reflection.

D Endoscope pistoned forward to visualize anterior portion of posterior horn.

E Normal posterior horn and posterior compartment beyond.

F Tear of notch attachment of medial meniscus.

G Bucket-handle tear in notch. Frequently this is difficult for the uninitiated arthroscopist to diagnose, because meniscus mechanically interferes with penetration of joint.

H Remaining rim of meniscus in bucket-handle tear. Notice abnormal size and contour. Small meniscus indicates bucket-handle tear.

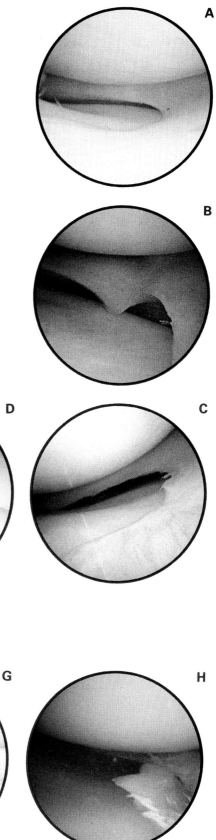

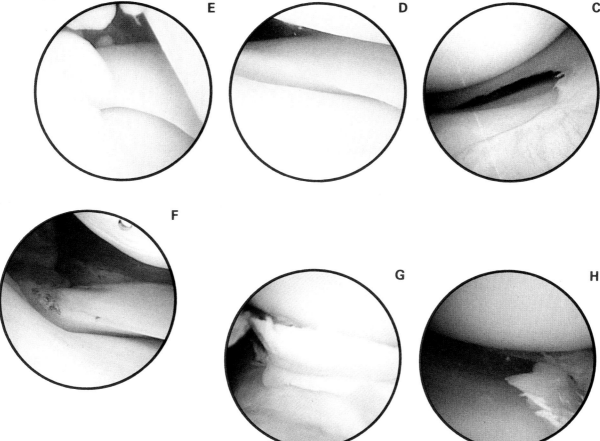

Posteromedial compartment

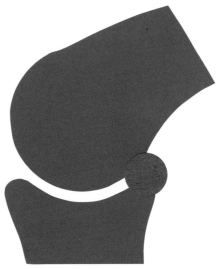

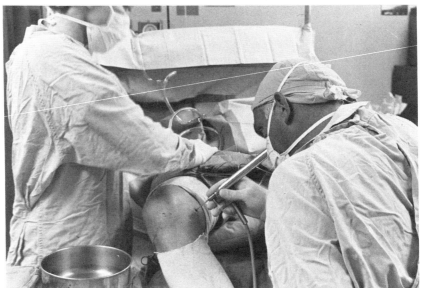

Patient The patient's thigh is allowed to roll into external rotation. The knee is flexed approximately 90°.

Assistant The assistant stabilizes the distal femur.

Physician The physician sits with the patient's foot in his lap. Arthroscopic approach is made from the posteromedial corner.

Maximal distention of the joint is essential to entry of the posteromedial compartment. Entry is posterior to the condyle and superior to the meniscus. Inspection of the compartment proceeds from the landmark junction of the femoral condyle and the meniscus.

The posterior cruciate ligament and the posterior horn of the medial meniscus can be visualized. In some patients, internal rotation of the tibia on the femur allows the meniscus to drop off the medial femoral condyle, making it possible to see vertical tears or abnormalities that would not be visible when the meniscus is resting against the femur. Retained posterior horns may be evaluated in this area.

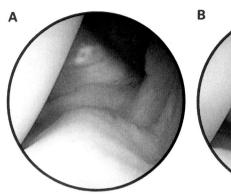

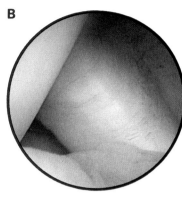

FIG. 7-6

A Posterior cruciate ligament seen just beyond junction of meniscus and femoral condyle.

B Close-up of normal posterior cruciate ligament in posteromedial compartment.

C Old separation of medial meniscus off posterior horn, not visible from front. No hemorrhage seen.

D Pistoning into cleft shows posterior tibial condyle deep in cleft.

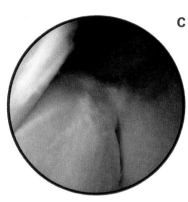

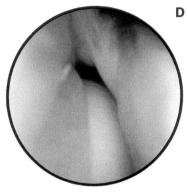

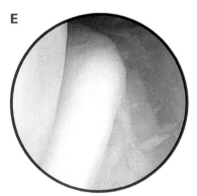

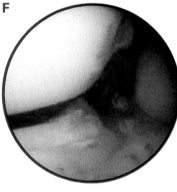

E Subacute posterior horn tear of medial meniscus.

F Acute posteromedial horn tear of meniscus, with hemorrhage in posterior capsule.

G Internal rotation of tibia on femur drops meniscus away from femur. Occult tears may be seen. Fronds of old anterior cruciate ligament tear were catching in joint.

H Retained posterior horn after anterovertical arthrotomy and removal of meniscus. There was second tear posterior to removed portion of meniscus. Retained posterior horn was torn off of its attachments, necessitating resection to reduce symptoms. Probably was an original untreated lesion.

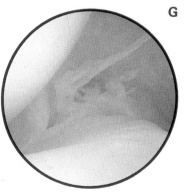

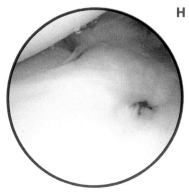

Posterolateral compartment

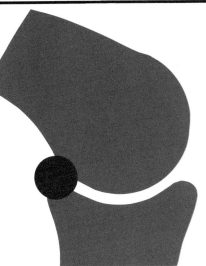

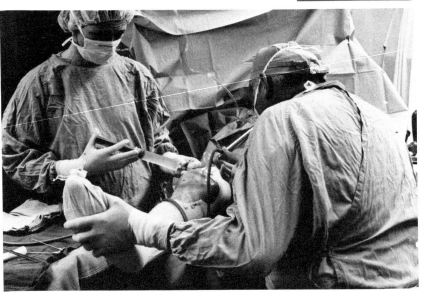

Patient   The patient is rolled slightly to the side of the uninvolved extremity. The knee is brought up into flexion of approximately 100°.

Assistant   The assistant is superior to the patient's side.

Physician   The physician stands next to the patient, with his foot on a stool rung and the patient's foot supported on his thigh.

The puncture is made at a point where a line drawn along the intermuscular septum intersects with a line drawn from the posterior aspect of the fibula. The endoscope is directed slightly anteroinferiorly to enter the posterolateral compartment. The junction between the meniscus and the articular surface can be visualized. Often the popliteus tendon is demonstrated as it enters the sheath posterolateral to the meniscus. Posterior horn tears not visible anteriorly are frequently identified, as is hemorrhagic change in the anterior cruciate ligament. Loose bodies collect in posterolateral compartment. There may be isolated tears of the anterior cruciate without any tear of the menisci. Invariably hemorrhage is seen within the posteromedial or posterolateral compartment, indicating an injury that cannot be documented clinically or arthroscopically from anterior puncture only.

FIG. 7-7

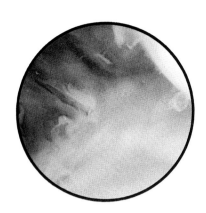

A Torn menisci not visible anteriorly are often seen in posterolateral compartment, especially in patients with torn ligamentous structures. If knee opened medially only, posterolateral tear of meniscus probably would be missed. Arthroscopic inspection allows design of surgical approach. Area cannot be visualized anteriorly even with small-diameter endoscope, because mass of meniscus blocks view.

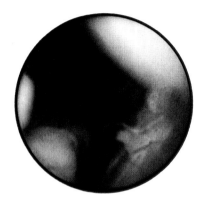

B Complete cleft in posterolateral meniscus.

C Posterolateral compartment collects many loose bodies and provokes rather marked degenerative synovitis. Methylene blue in joint for contrast.

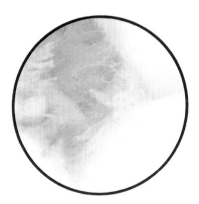

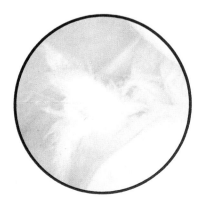

D Posterolateral puncture has been especially important in diagnosing anterior cruciate ligament injuries. Loose fragments of anterior cruciate tissue can be seen.

Chapter 8

Pathology

Pathologic arthroscopic findings
Meniscus in service of the articular cartilage
Condylar disease
Osteochondritis dissecans
Articular disease
Ligamentous injury
Synovial disease

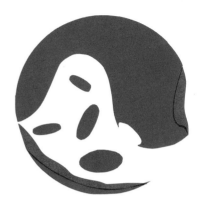

PATHOLOGIC ARTHROSCOPIC FINDINGS

The degenerative changes in menisci are mentioned in Chapter 7. The stage at which these become pathologic must be determined by interpretation of the patient's symptoms. Some patients have diffuse meniscal degeneration that is of little clinical significance because it is due to the aging process. Radiographically, juxtacortical increased densities may be apparent. Other patients have degenerative meniscal disease with large fragmentation or tears, which accelerates the degenerative process within a compartment.

Pathologic inspection of a cross section of menisci shows degenerative changes within the meniscal substance and a cleft separation between collagen fibers[2] (Fig. 8-1). A virgin meniscus does not tear in its substance. However, it is possible for it to tear off of its synovial attachment (see Fig. 9-2, *A* and *B*) without there being degenerative changes within the meniscal substance itself.

Arthroscopically, the earliest sign of degeneration of a meniscus is that the inner border loses its opaque nature and becomes translucent (Fig. 8-1, *A*). Arthroscopically it appears as though one is looking through ground glass.

This inner border can fragment and produce irregularities known as fringe tags (Figs. 8-1, *B*, and 8-2, *A*). These are asymptomatic. The small pieces that fragment out are cleaned by the synovial fluid and absorbed in the synovium.

A translucent inner border may separate from the body of the meniscus and appear as a fringe tear (Figs. 8-1, *C*, and 8-2, *B*). This particular lesion can mimic catching in or popping of the joint, often associated with a torn meniscus. In addition it can produce a positive McMurray sign. Such a lesion is very difficult to identify during surgery, because the knee has been dried; nor is magnification by arthroscopy or floating of the fringe tag in a fluid medium advantageous in identification. Many patients with positive physical findings of a torn meniscus but no lesion confirmed at surgery have been given meniscectomies "anyhow." They probably had fringe-type lesions. Obviously the symptoms are eliminated by total meniscectomy. However, these lesions need no surgical treatment; they are absorbed by the synovium, and the patient becomes asymptomatic.

Further evidence of degeneration is a cleft tear (Figs. 8-1, *D*, and 8-2, *C*). This may be a parrot-beak separation or a complete separation of the meniscus through its substance, forming a bucket-handle tear. This is the manifestation of deep interstitial fragmentation that has completely given way to stress.

A few patients examined arthroscopically for positive meniscal symptoms, including instability, have had normal findings. On repeat examination because of persistent symptoms for 4 to 6 months, a torn meniscus became apparent. There probably was a cleft tear deep in the meniscal surface or skin, which was not seen by the arthroscopist because it had not broken through the skin; yet fragmentation deep in the meniscus produced symptoms. Arthroscopy with local anesthetic allows repeat examination of these patients with ease and low risk. Therefore, we believe that meniscectomy should not be performed in the absence of definitive arthroscopic evidence.

Some patients have complete degenerative meniscal disease with large fragmentation tears that accelerate the degenerative process within the compartment (Fig. 8-2, *D*). This particular type of degeneration can be interrupted by meniscectomy. Even in the presence of substantial compartment loss, the knee can be improved. If these patients have tibia vara, tibial osteotomy may be considered. Gross disruption of the meniscus affecting the articular surface is also an indication for meniscectomy.

Arthroscopic observation of degenerative meniscal disease has added to our understanding of the management of meniscal abnormalities.

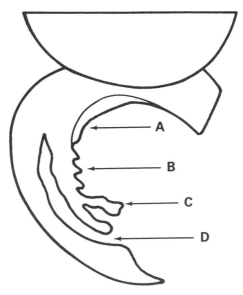

FIG. 8-1. *A,* Translucent inner border is first sign of degeneration of meniscus. *B,* Fringe tags occur when some translucent area sloughs off. *C,* Fringe tags or elevations of translucent inner degeneration may catch in joint and mimic positive McMurray sign. *D,* Cleft tears or complete tears within meniscus can occur when separations between collagen bundles completely separate.

FIG. 8-2

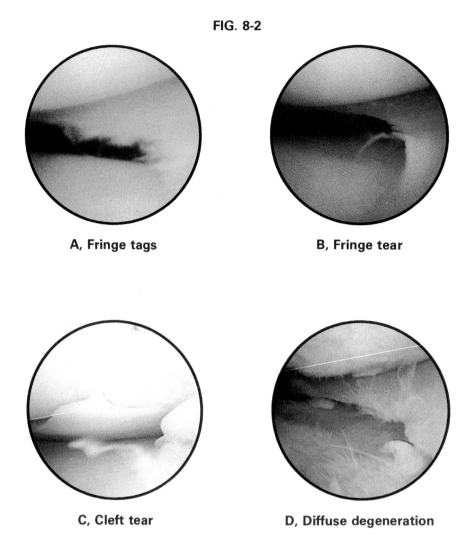

A, Fringe tags

B, Fringe tear

C, Cleft tear

D, Diffuse degeneration

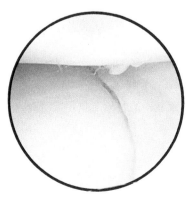

E, Regenerated meniscus after total meniscectomy.

MENISCUS IN SERVICE OF THE ARTICULAR CARTILAGE

The importance of the meniscus has been well established;[1] it is in service of the articular cartilage. Some peripheral detachment or hypermobility of the meniscus is not an indication for removal unless the meniscus tear, degeneration, or motion is doing a disservice to the adjacent articular cartilage. Symptoms that interfere with the patient's job or life style may also justify meniscectomy in a chronic peripherally detached meniscus in the absence of articular cartilage injury. However, unless the meniscus is violating the articular cartilage as demonstrated arthroscopically, the patient is best off without meniscectomy if the symptoms are tolerable.

The ease and safety of arthroscopy with local anesthetic allows monitoring by repeat examination. The effects of the meniscus on the articular cartilage can be determined before permanent findings of articular cartilage injury are manifest by roentgenographic changes.

CONDYLAR DISEASE

Arthroscopy provides a method of study of condylar disease and its treatment in patients with articular cartilage defects (see Fig. 11-1, *D*). Such defects may be traumatically or surgically produced. We have followed up on patients who have had drilling procedures on fragmented and fissured patellar surfaces and have observed curettage and drilling procedures on the femoral condyle. Articular defects of up to 2 cm in diameter will generally heal with vascular fibrous tissue in 6 weeks; by 12 weeks there will be a complete fibrocartilage replacement devoid of a vascular base, and the patient may commence increased physical activity. Arthroscopy provides direct vascular monitoring of the tissue healing.

In larger defects of up to 5 cm in diameter, it takes as long as 6 to 12 months to obtain articular healing sufficient to bear weight. Following and monitoring these defects with arthroscopy with local anesthetic shows that the active healing as visualized arthroscopically correlates very well with the clinical signs of decreased heat and inflammation.

OSTEOCHONDRITIS DISSECANS

In osteochondritis dissecans there is no correlation between symptoms and separation of the articular surfaces. The unseparated lesion can be monitored while treating with cast immobilization. Most defects heal in 6 months. Osteochondritis dissecans can be followed clinically in conjunction with arthroscopy with local anesthetic. The examination is enhanced by instillation of methylene blue for contrast (see Fig. 11-1, *A* and *B*).

ARTICULAR DISEASE

It is not unusual to observe articular injury or degeneration from articular disease arthroscopically prior to surgery. Articular disease worsens prognosis. Defects in the compartment opposite that with the major suspected pathologic abnormality have been seen that would probably have gone unnoticed in the absence of arthroscopy or a unicompartmental arthrotomy. These defects require curettage, elevation, or debridement of the articular cartilage or drilling to vascular bone.

Fissuring clefts accompany patellar dislocations. Rather than shaving these patellar clefts, multiple 1-mm holes are drilled in each cleft. Repeat arthroscopic inspection at 4 months shows sealing over of these clefts, and the patient becomes relatively asymptomatic. It may be possible to manage selected articular disease without complete debridement or shaving, which often does not provide the best long-term results.

LIGAMENTOUS INJURY

A number of patients have had intraligamentous hemorrhage that would have gone unnoticed without arthroscopy. This is commonly seen with rotation injury to the knee and hemarthrosis. Arthroscopic examination shows no separation of either menisci. There is a so-called isolated anterior cruciate tear without disruption of the synovium (see Fig. 12-1, A). It may be hemorrhagic throughoul its entirety, indicating the tear. Blood may disseminate through the adjacent subsynovial tissues in the intercondylar notch or into the fat pad. It should be noted that the so-called isolated anterior cruciate injuries universally show at least posteromedial and posterolateral capsular hemorrhage in the absence of posterior meniscal tears, but not to the extent that surgical repair is indicated. An isolated anterior cruciate injury is really a gross determination and does not reflect the diffuse disruption within the capsular tissues. Initially the knee may appear stable, but may become lax with time.

Some tears of the tibial collateral ligament are seen only intra-articularly. The patient has tenderness in the area but no palpable defect in the ligament. There is a synovial spearation above the meniscus or hemorrhagic changes such that the tibial collateral ligament can be visualized from inside the joint. Tears and stretches of the popliteal tendon have been seen with hemorrhagic changes, but they do not require surgical repair.

In patients with previous capsular injury and scar, the cannula and trocar meet more resistance during capsular penetration. It is a well-known principle of hand surgery that scar about the small joints and gliding tissues of the hand can be an impairment to function. The same is so of the knee joint but has not been given the same emphasis.

SYNOVIAL DISEASE

Synovial characteristics of aging show a gradual articular degenerative process. Small flakes of articular cartilage appear arthroscopically as stardust (Fig. 8-3, A), producing diffuse villous synovitis. Large loose bodies are easily seen (Fig. 8-3, B). Substantial synovial morphologic alterations occur in degenerative changes with loose articular pieces. The synovium eventually engulfs the articular cartilage (Fig. 8-3, C), but it may be removed through the arthroscopic cannula (Fig. 8-3, D). Because a synovial fluid cell block allows diagnosis of intra-articular tissue disease, biopsy is not required (Fig. 8-3, E). Debridement reduces the synovial reactions of resultant edema, fibrosis, and capsular thickening. Synovial characteristics in various diseases will be elaborated on in Chapter 13.

FIG. 8-3

A
B

A Stardusting. Loose synovial and articular fragments seen in suprapatellar pouch with transillumination.

B Multiple loose bodies between tibia and femur in medial compartment. Methylene blue enhances visualization.

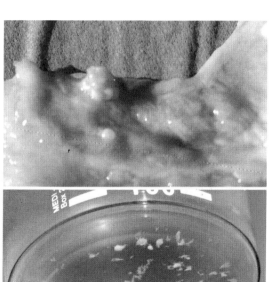

C Articular cartilage is engulfed by synovium if not removed from joint. May produce thickened synovium and capsule.

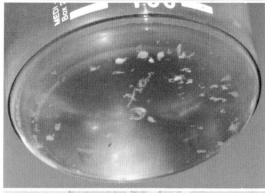

D Loose bodies vacuumed from joint through cannula.

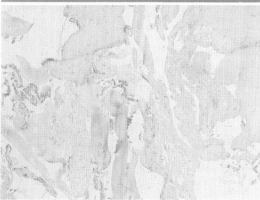

E Photomicrograph of synovial fluid cell block, including articular cartilage of synovial debris.

REFERENCES

1. Krause, W., Pope, M. N., Johnson, R., Weinstein, A., and Wilder, D.: Mechanical changes in the knee, post meniscectomy, J. Bone Joint Surg. (Br.) **57**(4):570, 1957.
2. Noble, J., and Hamblen, D. L.: The pathology of the degenerative meniscus lesion, J. Bone Joint Surg. (Br.) **57**(2):180-186, 1975.

Chapter 9

Meniscal disease

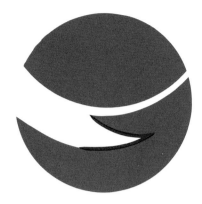

Normal meniscus
Torn meniscus
Degeneration of the meniscus
Peripheral detachment
Retained meniscus
Bucket-handle tear
Hypermobile meniscus
Postoperative evaluations

NORMAL MENISCUS

The meniscus is in service of the articular cartilage, and unless it is violating the articular cartilage, meniscectomy should be avoided. In some patients, peripherally detached menisci or cystic degeneration within the menisci produces symptoms such that meniscectomy is clinically indicated. Arthroscopy with local anesthetic has provided an easy and safe method of examining patients with knee problems thought to be meniscal abnormalities. Observation of meniscal degenerations and their concomitant natural history has prevented a number of unnecessary meniscectomies.

The posteromedial and posterolateral approaches have revealed a surprisingly high number of meniscal abnormalities not visible on anterior inspections of the joint (see Table 10, p. 81). Coexisting loose bodies in other compartments of the joint do not go unrecognized. Many can be managed arthroscopically by vacuuming the joint and thus avoiding a second arthrotomy. In some situations where there was certainty that an abnormality was located in a particular compartment of the joint, arthroscopy showed that it was either the opposite compartment that was involved or that there was a concomitant opposite compartment injury. The surgical plan was changed accordingly. Arthroscopy has saved patients unnecessary arthrotomy in areas where there was no meniscal abnormality. On the other hand, arthroscopy has revealed unsuspected lesions and has dictated an appropriate arthrotomy.

TORN MENISCUS

Arthroscopically there are four circumstantial signs of a torn meniscus (Fig. 9-1).

A normal meniscus has a sharp inner border, whereas an inner border that appears rounded off suggests a tear within the meniscus. A markedly rounded off meniscus is usually indicative of a bucket-handle tear.

The vertical and horizontal dimensions of the meniscus increase in size with degeneration. A large girth suggests a tear within the meniscus. Degeneration occurs first within the meniscal substance (Fig. 9-2, A). Breaking through of the clefts to the "skin" of the meniscus permits visualization of the tear.

Another circumstantial sign of a torn meniscus is a pile up of synovium around the synovial-meniscal reflection (Figs. 9-1 and 9-3, C). Normally transition is flat. If the meniscus is mobile and is catching and pulling off of its attachment, an exhaustive search for a meniscal tear should be made.

If the articular surface of the femur is roughened adjacent to the tibial spine, a tear of the posterior horn of the meniscus should be suspected (Fig. 9-1). This area will be localized and not diffuse. The condylar area is viewed with the knee in flexion. When the knee is extended, the area impinges on the posterior horn. When the tear is not visible anteriorly, it often can be identified by posterior puncture.

When any of these four signs exist, complete anterior and posterior inspections must be carried out in order to discover the torn meniscus.

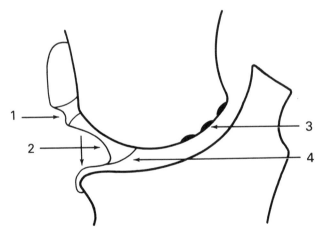

FIG. 9-1. Four circumstantial signs of torn meniscus. When any one is present arthroscopically, thorough search must be made for meniscal abnormality. *1,* Pile-up of synovium at meniscal-synovial reflection probably exists secondary to abnormal motion of meniscal attachment below. *2,* Increased anteroposterior or horizontal diameter of meniscus probably reflects interstitial separation of collagen bundles of meniscus. *3,* Localized area of degenerative arthritis adjacent to tibial spine suggests posterior horn tear of meniscus in that compartment. Separate posteromedial or posterolateral inspection is obligatory to rule out lesion not visualized anteriorly. *4,* Rounded off inner border of meniscus suggests either parrot-beak tear or old tear of meniscus.

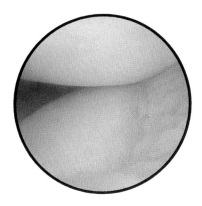

FIG. 9-2

A Pileup of synovium at the meniscal-synovial junction suggests a tear somewhere in the meniscus.

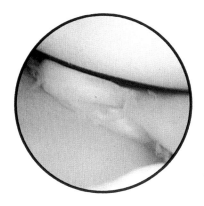

B Rounded inner border of the meniscus or thickening in vertical or horizontal dimension is a sign of a disruption of the meniscus.

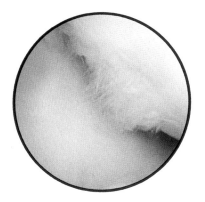

C Injured articular cartilage on the femoral condyle adjacent to the tibial spine alerts the arthroscopist to a posterior horn tear not seen from the anterior view.

FIG. 9-3

A Acute peripheral detachment of meniscus seen only by probing area adjacent to tibial collateral ligament. Photograph shows hemorrhagic change of peripheral tear, only seen with a valgus strain on knee and pistoning forward into this area.

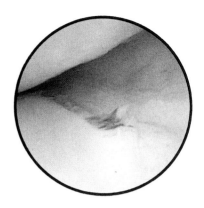

B Posteromedial inspection of peripheral detachment of meniscus, from posteromedial toward anterior. Tibial collateral ligament (light colored strip) to left. Methylene blue in joint for contrast. Peripheral tear of meniscus not seen from anterior, even with small-diameter endoscope, because very tight knee did not allow sufficient opening of medial compartment to inspect area.

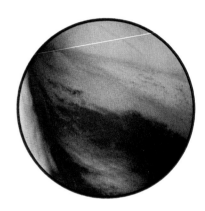

C Old peripheral detachments or tear of menisci evident by sulcus at synovial-meniscal reflection or buildup of synovium in area. Arthroscopic photograph shows sulcus at meniscal-synovial reflection. Lesion correlates well with patient's symptoms of pain and instability.

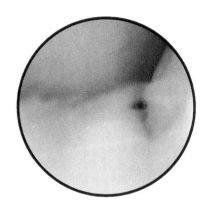

DEGENERATION OF THE MENISCUS

The stages of degeneration observed arthroscopically in the meniscus are outlined in Chapter 8. Fringe tears can mimic meniscal tears clinically (Fig. 9-2). These lesions, when identified arthroscopically, do not require surgical intervention; the synovial fluid cleanses them, and they are absorbed by the synovium, rendering the patient asymptomatic. It should be noted that this is an early sign of degeneration and that in later years a torn meniscus may develop, with separation of the collagen bundles.

Some patients have had clinical signs and symptoms of a torn meniscus but normal arthroscopic findings. Within 4 to 6 months, because of persistent symptoms, repeat arthroscopy carried out with local anesthetic showed a complete tear in an area easily visualized in the previous arthroscopic examination. It is my opinion that these patients had interstitial separations of the collagen bundles, with deformation of the meniscus causing the symptoms. Because the lesion had not broken through the surface of the meniscus, it was not visualized arthroscopically. It would not have been seen on an arthrogram either, because there was no separation of the meniscus for the dye to move into.

We have observed patients with meniscal symptoms and deformation of the meniscus but no complete tears. This is especially noticed in the posteromedial and posterolateral horns of the menisci. Meniscectomy is unnecessary if the symptoms are tolerable. In those patients who choose meniscectomy for symptomatic reasons, I have seen marked degeneration in the area of the deformation. Undoubtedly the meniscus had undergone previous injury without complete separation. It should be restated that every effort should be made to discourage meniscectomy unless the articular surface is injured.

PERIPHERAL DETACHMENT

An acute peripheral detachment is easily identified (Fig. 9-3, *A*). It is important to inspect the area of the meniscal-synovial reflection in acute injuries. In hyperextension injury, the separation can be off the anterior horn. In some rotational injuries, especially with a torn anterior cruciate ligament, the area at the tibial collateral ligament will have a separation of approximately ½ to 1 inch in length, which can only be visualized with penetration of the endoscope into this area while valgus stress is applied.

In some patients no meniscal injury was visible anteriorly and the diagnosis was substantiated by posterior inspection. The separation was not seen initially with posterior puncture but only with slow retraction of the endoscope and angulation toward the tibial collateral ligament (Fig. 9-3, *B*). This again emphasizes the importance of posterior inspections. The same has been so for the posterolateral corner near the attachment of the popliteus tendon, because it goes through its synovial sheath posteriorly and laterally to the lateral meniscus. Peripheral detachments are not necessarily accompanied by degeneration of the meniscus.

Suturing of peripheral tears results in further attenuation and articular injury in young people, because they are active. I have attempted to allow peripheral detachments in adolescents to heal themselves. They will seal down in a couple of months, but they remain painful and attenuated. If patients are very active, they are prone to complete tears within the next several months[1] (Fig. 9-3, *C*).

The ability to inspect these peripheral lesions arthroscopically encouraged me to treat patients in their early teens conservatively. My clinical impression that peripheral detachments would seal down and become asymptomatic has not been borne out, and existing clefts with synovial proliferation along the medial meniscus have been easily identified. Therefore, when there is peripheral detachment of the meniscus, except perhaps in selected circumstances, meniscectomy at the time of the injury reduces overall morbidity.

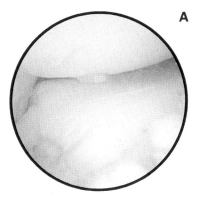

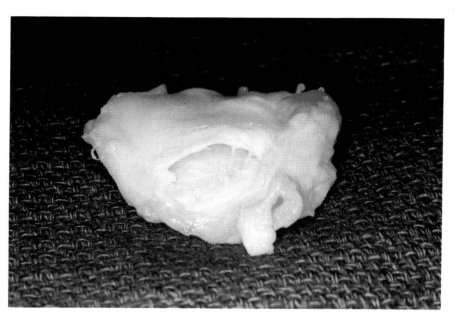

FIG. 9-4. A, Discoid meniscus usually fills entire compartment, most often laterally. Frequently symptomatic. Although tear may not be seen arthroscopically, horizontal cleft tears commonly produce symptoms. **B,** Discoid meniscus, gross anatomy. Photograph shows degeneration and horizontal cleft tear within discoid meniscus. Lesion would not have been identified arthroscopically because it had not broken through skin of meniscus, nor would it be identified by arthrogram; yet it was symptomatic, producing complaints of instability.

RETAINED MENISCUS

Patients have been referred to me for arthroscopic evaluation because symptoms persisted after short anterovertical arthrotomy for resection of the meniscus. A typical syndrome includes a partial tear of the anterior cruciate ligament, a short anterovertical arthrotomy, and a retained posterior meniscus. Histologic sections show that this is not a regenerated meniscus but actually an incompletely excised posterior horn. The medial compartment is most commonly affected. When these retained menisci are long standing in the presence of mild instability, degenerative changes are virtually always present, frequently manifested by the presence of loose bodies. Many of these patients had a tear of the posterolateral meniscus that was not identified at the time of arthrotomy but could have been seen had a comprehensive arthroscopy been carried out prior to surgery.

For the past 10 years I have ascribed to meniscectomy carried out at the level of vascularity, that is, complete meniscectomy of all degenerative meniscal tissue. This is based on the fact that a torn meniscus is not a virgin lesion but a result of previous trauma and degeneration of the collagen fibers. I have seen patients who have had subtotal meniscectomies, yet had three vertical tears in the posterior retained meniscus, as well as patients who have had bucket-handle tears removed, yet had as many as two subsequent bucket-handle tears in the remaining degenerative meniscal tissue. My arthroscopic experience with patients on whom subtotal meniscectomy had been performed by other physicians has universally shown progressive degeneration of the meniscus or compartment, with irregular meniscal tissue. However, arthroscopic 10-year follow-up studies on patients with complete meniscectomies, through both anterior and posterior arthrotomies, show no progressive degeneration or compartment collapse.

Meniscectomy done at the level of vascularity allows regeneration of fibrous tissue. Meniscectomy done in the absence of vascularity allows only the irregular inner border of the degenerative meniscus to persist.

Resection of a retained posterior meniscus will alleviate the symptoms if degenerative changes or loose bodies do not exist. When a retained meniscus is accompanied by rotary instability or loss of the cruciate ligament and medial supporting structures, resection of the posterior horn with a reconstructive procedure is indicated to reduce the progressive morbidity.

BUCKET-HANDLE TEAR

One of the difficult lesions for the uninitiated arthroscopist to identify is the bucket-handle tear. Clinically, diagnosis is simple. Arthroscopically, because the mass of the meniscus is in the intercondylar notch, it interferes frequently with the penetration of the endoscope and blocks the view. After seeing a few bucket-handle tears in the notch, their diagnosis becomes easier. Some patients with a complete bucket-handle tear that is all the way in the notch will not have the usual lack of range of motion, making clinical diagnosis difficult.

The posterior meniscal separations are perpendicular to the articular surfaces of the tibia and therefore are not visible anteriorly. It should be noted that in the presence of a torn anterior cruciate ligament or a ligamentous injury related to the medial compartment, the frequency of the occult posteromedial or posterolateral meniscal tear increases. Therefore, whenever a completely or incompletely torn cruciate ligament is identified, potential posterolateral and posteromedial meniscal separations should be suspected. Therefore, posterior puncture techniques are encouraged.

HYPERMOBILE MENISCUS

Many patients have had meniscectomies for so-called hypermobile menisci. Arthroscopy has provided an opportunity to evaluate this condition and discern that there is no underlying tear within the meniscus. I have seen menisci that were clinically hypermobile and have confirmed the diagnosis at arthroscopy with manipulation of the knee. Attenuation of the coronary ligaments can allow the meniscus to become increasingly mobile and symptomatic. This can occur in patients who have normally hypermobile joints; the increased natural laxity of the joint allows increased mobility of the menisci. Unless the meniscus is injuring the articular surface, I advise against meniscectomy. The abnormality should be explained to the patient, and he should be assured that he does not have a meniscal tear or articular cartilage damage. Most patients will accept the diagnosis and modify their activities accordingly, thus avoiding meniscectomy.

POSTOPERATIVE EVALUATIONS

Postoperative evaluations are most commonly asked for in those patients who have had a meniscectomy through a short anterovertical approach. These patients have retained posterior horns of the meniscus, most often with concomitant degenerative condylar changes or loose bodies.

I have observed patients who have had a complete arthroscopic examination and medial meniscectomy, who during the 8 to 10 weeks after surgery have incurred a relatively minor knee injury with meniscal symptoms in the opposite compartment. I was hesitant to believe there was anything more than a tear of fibrous tissue; however, in several patients a second tear of the meniscus has been observed this early in the postoperative course. Therefore, any patient who has undergone a meniscectomy, but who has any meniscal symptoms postoperatively or slow rehabilitation, is a candidate for arthroscopy with local anesthetic to evaluate the intra-articular status.

These evaluations have shown that synovitis following arthrotomy is usually subsequent to degenerative arthritis with fine debris in the joint (see Chapter 8). Unexplained synovitis following arthrotomy is a clear indication for arthroscopy, at which time the existence of any other articular abnormality can be identified. Most often there are loose bodies in the joint, which can be vacuumed out during arthroscopy, avoiding morbidity and prolonged rehabilitation.

The theory that synovitis is secondary to lack of patient initiative in progressive quadriceps exercises has been dismissed. In fact, arthroscopic inspection after arthrotomy shows that patients who are rehabilitated with vigorous and almost abusive progressive quadriceps exercise universally develop degeneration of the patellofemoral articulation with loose bodies. This most often occurs if activity is initiated within 6 weeks after surgery. During this time the articular surfaces are most succulent and more prone to injury due to compressive and shearing forces during heavy progressive quadriceps exercises. For this reason, I have restrained patients in the healing phases from that type of activity and have initiated isometric quadriceps exercises until there is maturation of the fibrous tissue and no inflammatory signs about the joint. Then increased activity is certainly safe.

In a number of patients who erroneously were instructed or believed that the joint would heal faster with exercise, condylar injury or loose bodies have resulted. Thus I instruct patients to let the wound heal first; then work for range of motion and isometric strength; and then, following maturation and healing, work for increased power.

REFERENCE

1. Schneider, D. A., and Johnson, L. L.: Peripheral detachment of the meniscus: arthroscopic evaluation and clinical correlation, Orthop. Rev., September 1977.

Patellar disease

Arthroscopy has confirmed the clinical diagnosis in a high percentage of patients with patellar conditions, as opposed to meniscal lesions, which have a rather low incidence of exact correlation (see Tables 2, 6, and 7, pp. 76, 79, and 80). Patellar conditions are relatively straightforward. However, some conditions clinically interpreted as torn menisci or torn ligaments have been arthroscopically established as patellar abnormalities.

The patella can be viewed in most patients through an anteromedial puncture. Very gentle retraction of the endoscope is necessary to bring the patella into tangential view. If there is any compromise in the inspection from below, due to obesity, scar tissue, or osteophytes on the patella, an auxillary suprapatellar examination is indicated (see Fig. 3-33). If the patella is at all suspect as the primary site of abnormality, a suprapatellar examination is routine. If a dislocation of the patella is suspected, inspection from above is from the lateral side. Routinely, the patella is inspected from the medial side because it is technically easier. With the patient's thigh in external rotation, the patellofemoral articulation can be viewed from above. It is possible to see the undersurface of the patella, the suprapatellar pouch, and the fat pad.

With the patient under local anesthesia, dynamics of the knee joint can be observed while the patient contracts the quadriceps mechanism or by flexion and extension. An artifact is produced by distention of the capsule from saline in the joint. Therefore, interpretations of patellar gliding are not completely valid. It should be noted that during quadriceps compression, the tongue of the fat pad moves proximally under the patella. It is unusual for this to be symptomatic when palpated with the endoscope with use of local anesthetic or during quadriceps compression.

Endoscopic palpation of the patellar surface can be carried out with local anesthesia. Correlation of pain in this area may duplicate the patient's prearthroscopic complaints.

CHONDROMALACIA

Many patients are thought clinically to have chondromalacia of the patella (Fig. 10-1), because their pain is in the area of the patella or because with flexion and extension they have crepitus in the kneecap. They may complain of pain while walking up and down stairs or after prolonged sitting. The physical examination may produce pain in the patellar area, with quadriceps tightening against resistance applied to the patella.

Chondromalacia of the patella is a common diagnosis arthroscopically, but not every patient who has the above symptoms has chondromalacia (i.e., many young girls who have no pathologic abnormality and an absolutely smooth patella).

In those patients who have some symptoms of chondromalacia as well as pain referred to the medial joint line, the differential diagnosis can be challenging. Arthroscopic examination with local anesthetic establishes the diagnosis. Most frequently, patients with the above-mentioned symptom complex and medially referred pain have chondromalacia patellae. Only a few have a torn meniscus, and some have loose bodies throughout the joint (Figs. 10-1 to 10-3). These can be vacuumed out, reducing the symptoms.

Confirmation of the diagnosis by arthroscopic direct visualization increases the physician's confidence in a conservative treatment program and engenders acceptance on the part of the patient or the patient's parents.

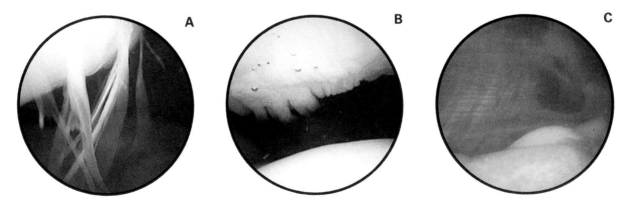

FIG. 10-1. **A,** Chondromalacia of patella, bacon-strip type. Filmy articular strips can come off patella, especially at superior pole. These frequently are free in joint. Compare with Fig. 10-2. **B,** Chondromalacia of patella, with saw-tooth type appearance of shaggy loose articular cartilage. **C,** Progression under patella into suprapatellar pouch shows normal synovium except for some minimal hemosiderin staining. Notice flattened wall and lack of villae in this relatively nonreactive tissue.

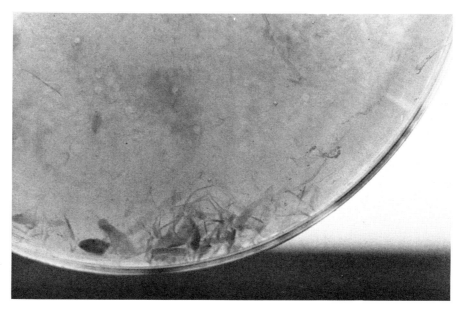

FIG. 10-2. Loose articular fragments off of patella, such as seen in Fig. 10-1, *A.*

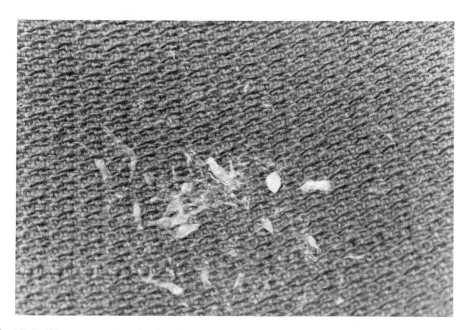

FIG. 10-3. Close-up of articular fragments strained onto towel for closer observation. Material must be absorbed by joint, producing discomfort.

DISLOCATION

Dislocation of the patella is to be suspected in virtually any injury of the knee (Fig. 10-4). In a series of patients, ligamentous and torn menisci were suspected prearthroscopically, but the defects of dislocation of the patella were observed at the time of inspection of the joint. Arthroscopy has increased my suspicion that patellar conditions mimic meniscal or ligamentous abnormalities.

A defect in the lateral femoral condyle may be identified arthroscopically (Fig. 10-4, *B*). A piece of bone may be knocked out of this area in acute dislocations of the patella. The loose body invariably is in the lateral sulcus and is engulfed by the synovium in a couple of weeks. Occasionally there can be a patellar injury with acute dislocation of the patella (Fig. 10-4, *C*). Lateral joint tenderness may mimic a torn lateral meniscus.

Arthroscopy with local anesthetic is of special value in confirming a diagnosis of acute dislocation of the patella and dictating the appropriate treatment. The presence or absence of loose bodies can be established. Many articular injuries do not involve enough bone to show up well on roentgenograms, and even when a large loose body is involved, the x-ray examination may be compromised because of the patient's discomfort. Acute dislocation of the patella with a chunk of articular cartilage in the joint increases morbidity and prolongs rehabilitation. In some patients under local anesthesia, we have elected to remove the loose body arthroscopically with a Jaws modified pituitary ronjeur. In others, the extent of the soft-tissue tear was so evident that we recommended surgical repair.

At surgery for chronic dislocations of the patella, the articular defect can be seen over the lateral femoral condyle, with depression and abrasion of the surface. There may also be loose bodies in the posterior compartment; thus, posterolateral inspection is important to their detection and removal. In addition, concomitant torn anterior cruciate ligaments and torn menisci may be seen in recurrent dislocation of the patella.

The lesion in the lateral femoral condyle is in a surprisingly low position on that condyle. The knee must be in approximately 90° flexion for the depression or articular fracture to occur with patellar dislocation. Therefore, during physical examination of the patient it is important that the test for hypermobile patella or dislocation of the patella be done with the knee at 90° flexion rather than complete extension. Some patients who in no way have clinical dislocations of the patella have very mobile patellae in complete extension, because the quadriceps expansion is taut in flexion. Other patients have no suggestion of mobility in the extended position or even a particularly high-riding patella; yet when the knee is brought down to 90° flexion and force is applied to move the patella laterally, they will grimace, confirming the presence of acute dislocation.

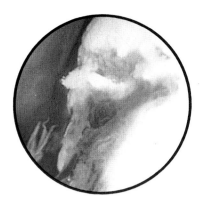

FIG. 10-4. Acute dislocation of patella.

A Hemorrhagic defect of articular fracture as seen in tangential view of lateral femoral condyle. This is usually one finger breadth superior and lateral to lateral meniscal-synovial reflection.

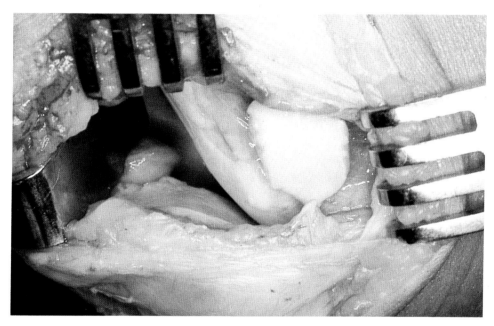

B Defect of lateral femoral condyle at time of surgery. Articular fragment engulfed in synovium laterally on lateral femoral condyle. Notice that knee is in 90° flexion in order for patella to shift out in this area.

C Arthroscopic view of same patellar defect.

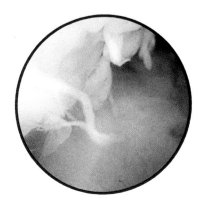

SUBLUXATION

Subluxation of the patella is a common and frequently unsuspected abnormality. Review of my series shows that in a number of patients articular defects and depression of the lateral femoral condyle suggested a diagnosis of patellar subluxation long before it was clinically suspected. In addition, potential subluxation of the patella may be suspected in girls with knee symptoms, especially patellar, but no clinical evidence of a defect in the lateral femoral condyle. In a number of such patients in whom arthroscopic findings were normal, subluxation was confirmed within a year. Patients should be advised to watch for the manifestation.

ACUTE FRACTURE

Arthroscopy can be of benefit in diagnosis of an acute fracture of the patella. It may not be possible to establish by x-ray examination the amount of separation or displacement of the patellar surfaces. Arthroscopy with local anesthetic can establish the amount of disruption of tissue. Frequently there is an alteration of the articular surface not seen on the roentgenogram, and there may be loose articular pieces in the joint that can only be identified and removed arthroscopically.

Not every fractured patella need be examined arthroscopically, but there are those selected cases where it can be of benefit in planning treatment.

OLD FRACTURES

Some patients with old fractures of the patella have benefited from arthroscopic examination. It has been possible to establish complete union of the articular surfaces or an existing chondromalacia of the patella at the fracture line. It is not uncommon to have symptomatic fragmentation of articular surfaces at the area where even a moderately displaced patellar fracture existed.

Some patients have been arthroscopically evaluated for medicolegal purposes.

OSTEOCHONDRITIS DISSECANS

Osteochondritis dissecans can be determined by arthroscopic examination. It is difficult to tell whether the lesion has separated or whether there is a bone abnormality without articular separation. Arthroscopy with methylene blue stain can establish the integrity of the articular surface. If the articular surface is loose, excision may be indicated. We have seen one case of osteochondritis dissecans of the patella with a loose body in the posterolateral compartment. Had it not been detected through posterolateral puncture, synovitis would have resulted until the loose body was completely absorbed.

RUPTURED TENDON

Some patients have dysfunction of the knee secondary to either a new or old ruptured quadriceps or patellar tendon. It is especially important in reconstructive surgery to assess the entire intra-articular status of the joint. If no abnormality is detected by arthroscopy within the joint, arthrotomy is not indicated, and repair of the tendon can proceed, with surgery limited to the lesion itself. The fibrosis from extended surgery is avoided, and the rehabilitation time is shortened.

CONTUSION OF THE KNEE

I have seen patients who had direct blows to the area of the knee, with resultant hemarthroses or suspected articular fracture of the patella. A direct blow to the synovium against the end of the femur can produce a hematoma and effusion, which can mimic a ligamentous injury. There is decreased range of motion. The diagnosis is easily established arthroscopically, and the appropriate conservative rehabilitation measures can be instituted.

It is possible that a direct blow to the patella will not fracture the osseous substance but only the articular surface. Diffuse stellate bursting fractures of the articular surface, with considerable morbidity have been seen in athletes who have fallen on hard surfaces. There was no evidence of articular fracture. Debridement of the articular material shortened rehabilitation.

POSTOPERATIVE EVALUATION
Patella baja

Postoperative evaluations have been carried out in patients with patella baja who have had aggressive Hauser reconstruction of the knee with considerable pain. One of the causes of pain following an aggressive Hauser procedure may be compression of the fat pad between the patella and the tibia; subtotal resection may give relief of symptoms. In one patient with mild chondromalacia of the patella, a recess of the plug of bone resulted in remission of symptoms, and patellectomy was not indicated. Another patient had only minimal chondromalacia of the distal pole of the patella and a rather large fat pad. An arthrotomy was carried out. The screw was removed from the tibia; the fat pad, which was massive and compressed in the intercondylar notch, was excised; and the roughened distal pole of the patella was shaved. This rendered the patient asymptomatic.

Metallic prosthesis

Complications have been seen in patients with metallic patellar prostheses. One patient had marked chondromalacia of the intercondylar notch, with pain on palpation in that area; removal of the prosthesis was recommended. A second patient had a painful knee without chondromalacia on the intercondylar notch; further conservative treatment was suggested.

Subtotal patellectomy

Evaluation of a variety of subtotal patellectomies has shown that the remaining articular surface was markedly fragmented and degenerated, that there was tilting of the patella in the junction between the patella and the patellar surfaces, or that the surfaces were irregular and symptomatic. Definitive treatment can only be based on arthroscopic evaluation of the pathologic findings.

Patellectomy

Some patients who have had patellectomies have complained of pain or catching in the area of the arthrotomy or the site of the anastomosis of the quadriceps and patellar tendon. In one patient a rather large piece of tissue was hanging from the anastomosis, causing it to catch in the joint during extension and flexion. Excision of the large mass of tissue rendered the patient asymptomatic. The diagnosis could not be established other than by arthroscopy.

BIPARTITE PATELLA

Most patients with bipartite patella and symptoms have no chondromalacia or articular separation in the area of the defect. Sometimes a differential diagnosis between the fracture and bipartite patella can only be confirmed arthroscopically.

In two patients with x-ray evidence of bipartite patella, severe pain over years was managed conservatively without benefit. Arthroscopic examination showed marked chondromalacia at the junction of the nonunion site. A subsequent arthrotomy and excision of the extra ossicle, which in fact was a nonunion site all the way through the articular surface, gave remission of symptoms.

PARAPATELLAR SYNOVITIS

In parapatellar synovitis, long villae of synovium, very much like fringe, surround the patella. These synovial tags are not rheumatoid but degenerative in morphologic character. They can catch between the patella and femoral surfaces, and often the tips hemorrhage and swell. Universal remission of symptoms has been achieved with conservative treatment, including isometric exercise and salicylates. Parapatellar synovitis is one anatomical explanation for knee discomfort in young girls.

Chapter 11

Condylar disease

Fractures
Degenerative changes
Loose bodies
Degenerative synovitis
Osteochondritis dissecans
Osteochondral defects
Preoperative evaluations
Postoperative evaluations

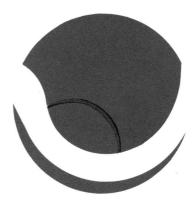

Arthroscopy provides a method of observation of the articular cartilage not available by any other method. By the time a roentgenogram shows juxta-articular hypertrophic bony changes, articular cartilage disease is usually far advanced. Still the x-ray examination does not reveal whether there is regenerated articular surface, complete loss of articular surface, or raw ebonated bone. The presence or absence of most loose bodies cannot be identified except by arthroscopy.

FRACTURES

The existence of an intra-articular fracture of the knee joint with ligamentous injury can be determined by arthroscopy. Inspection of the joint can establish the amount of displacement and the presence or absence of concomitant intra-articular ligamentous or meniscal tears. For example, if a patient has a medial plateau fracture with displacement sufficient to warrant reduction by open surgery, there may be an accompanying lateral compartment tear or cruciate ligament tear. The amount of surgical dissection necessary to reduce the fracture can be limited by knowledge obtained arthroscopically. The meniscus need not be unnecessarily removed to reduce an intra-articular fracture. In a fracture where radiologic findings secondary to magnification are overread, arthroscopy can demonstrate that the separation is minimal. Surgery is avoided, and casting is all that is required.

DEGENERATIVE CHANGES

Degeneration of the articular cartilage can vary from early bacon-strip fragmentation, as seen in the patella (see Fig. 10-1), to convolutions. Further degeneration will show exposed yellow bone (Fig. 11-2). The synovium in degenerative arthritis can be acutely inflamed (see Chapter 9) or there can be a very fine filamentous degenerative change, especially in the posterolateral compartment.

At the present time the main value of arthroscopy in degenerative arthritic disease is in establishing the exact status of the disease or in evaluating it from an investigative standpoint.

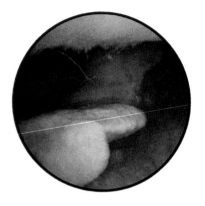

FIG. 11-1. Hypertrophic spurring on medial femoral condyle adjacent to patella in progressive degenerative arthritis.

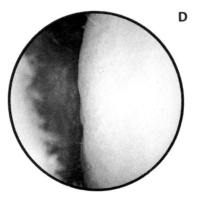
D

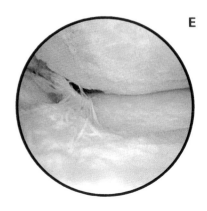
E

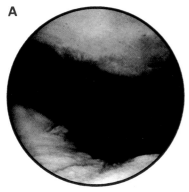
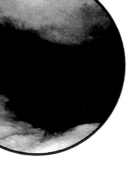

FIG. 11-2

A Composition shows motion involved in arthroscopy. Starting superiorly, view under patella and intercondylar notch. Juxta-articular surfaces are markedly degenerated.

B With slight retraction of endoscope, view now encompasses only intercondylar notch, with loss of articular surface. Methylene blue is in joint. Patella not seen.

C Farther down intercondylar notch, fat pad comes into view at left.

D Endoscope moved up tangential surface of femoral condyle. Synovial wall to left; articular surface of condyle at periphery has good regenerated cartilage.

E Inspection along lateral compartment shows complete degeneration of articular surfaces and degenerated torn meniscus.

F Absence of bone on medial femoral condyle, which appears yellow.

G Intercondylar notch shows degenerated synovial tissue over anterior cruciate ligament. No loose bodies.

H Entire medial compartment with degenerative meniscus and loss of articular surface on both femur and tibia.

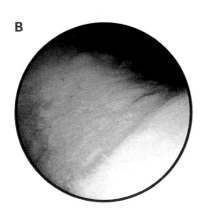

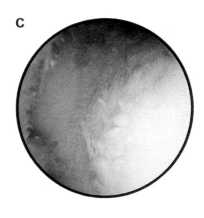

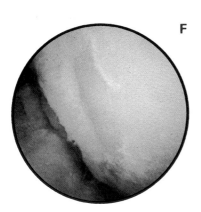

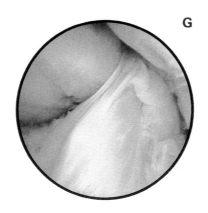

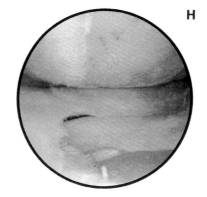

LOOSE BODIES

Loose bodies are more common than is clinically expected. The easy access to visualization of the joint by arthroscopy with the patient under local anesthesia, preceeding arthrotomy with general anesthesia, has shown a surprisingly high incidence of loose bodies. These often mimic other conditions, such as a torn meniscus. Many loose bodies can be managed arthroscopically, either by removing them with various sized cannulas and vacuuming (see Chapter 8) or by removing larger loose bodies with the Jaws modified pituitary ronjeur (see Fig. 11-3, A).

The natural course of loose bodies is for them to be absorbed in the synovium. In a patient with a large number of loose bodies, the synovium will actually engulf the articular material. A synovectomy may be indicated.

DEGENERATIVE SYNOVITIS

Acute nonarticular synovitis with considerable inflammation is representative of a rather acute degenerative process with multiple fine loose bodies in the joint. Arthroscopy and removal of these loose bodies reverses the process and renders the patient asymptomatic.

OSTEOCHONDRITIS DISSECANS

The management or investigation of osteochondritis dissecans is facilitated by arthroscopy (Fig. 11-3, B and C). In new patients with osteochondritis dissecans the usual procedure is to inspect the area of the defect with the patient under local anesthesia. Staining with methylene blue demonstrates whether the articular surface is intact. It is also possible to palpate the area and establish whether there is loosening or pain, which can affect management. If the defect is intact and painless, conservative treatment and immobilization will usually result in healing in 6 months. If the defect is small and loose, surgical removal is indicated, with sharp excision of the bed down to bleeding juxta-articular bone.

If a defect has not healed after a number of months, repeat arthroscopy with local anesthetic can be carried out.

OSTEOCHONDRAL DEFECTS

Defects of the articular surface of the knee can occur from trauma or surgery. In acute dislocations of the patella, loss of the articular surface of the lateral femoral condyle is common (see Fig. 10-2). Some patients lose large portions of the articular surface of the patella as well.

In patients with articular cartilage injuries, bucket-handle tears of the meniscus, or osteochondritis dissecans, a sharp surgical excision perpendicular to the articular surface is indicated for removal of the soft loose fragmented articular surface. Small lesions will heal within 6 weeks. Larger lesions (1 inch) may take 12 to 14 weeks before the vascularity of the bed of the lesion dissolves and becomes fibrocartilaginous. Restriction of weight-bearing activities until these defects have healed reduces morbidity. Healing, as seen arthroscopically, correlates well with the absence of inflammatory symptoms. (See Fig. 11-3, D.)

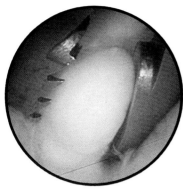

Osteochondritis dissecans.

FIG. 11-3

A Loose body in posteromedial compartment being removed by Jaws modified pituitary ronjeur.

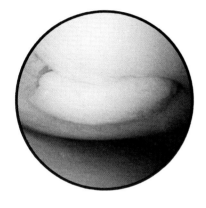

B Area of osteochondritis dissecans separated from articular surface.

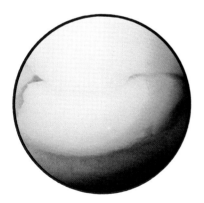

C Methylene blue can be advantageous in clearly delineating articular separation, especially in situations less subtle than this.

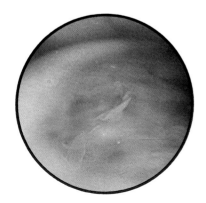

D Large defect created surgically down to raw bleeding bone, 6 weeks prior to this intra-articular photography.

PREOPERATIVE EVALUATIONS

Arthroscopy is potentially beneficial in evaluating tibial osteotomy or total-joint resurfacing, because it can verify the presence or absence of articular cartilage. Raw bone in a compartment, not yet manifested by roentgenographic changes, or a torn meniscus is probably a contraindication to shifting weight to the unaffected compartment. In the future, arthroscopy should provide a method of more refined selection of patients for tibial osteotomy. Evaluation of articular cartilage injury can show symptomatic hypertrophic osteophytes without marked change in the articular surface or meniscus. Patients with such injuries may be candidates for Magnusson "house cleaning" at the time of surgery.

Arthroscopic evaluation of a patient who is a candidate for so-called total-knee replacement can establish the presence or absence of articular surfaces. The necessity for unicompartmental or bicompartmental resurfacing may be reevaluated. Potentially, the existence of patellar disease could influence the decision to resurface or remove a patella.

POSTOPERATIVE EVALUATIONS

Violation of the articular cartilage is the most serious injury that the knee joint can undergo. Arthroscopic evaluation in patients who underwent surgery for an injury to meniscal or ligamentous tissue, but whose morbidity increased over the subsequent weeks and months, often show articular cartilage injury. Simple meniscal injury without evidence of articular cartilage injury at the time of surgery has been seen. Within 6 to 8 weeks, effusion and discomfort developed. Arthroscopic examination showed articular cartilage dissection off the femoral condyle. It is presumed that there was a shearing injury to the articular cartilage at the time of the meniscal injury, but that it was not evident at the time of arthrotomy because the articular cartilage was not vascular and the patient had a low metabolic rate. This injury was identified only by arthroscopy at a later date, and loose bodies were removed from the joint.

Chapter 12

Extrasynovial lesions

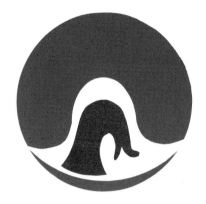

TORN LIGAMENTS
Anterior cruciate

A torn anterior cruciate ligament is a rather common injury (Fig. 12-1). It was present in 15% of 962 knees reviewed. It was a less common finding in the total patient population examined diagnostically under local anesthesia, but was seen in 30% of 162 consecutive knees of patients examined under general anesthesia over a 1-year period.

Diagnosis of a torn anterior cruciate ligament can be difficult clinically because of the existence of pain and hemarthrosis and resultant muscular guarding on the part of the patient. Unless there is an accompanying stretch of the lateral or medial supporting structures or gross instability of all structures, the presence of cruciate ligament injury can be masked.

The arthrogram is virtually totally inept as an aid in diagnosing torn anterior cruciate ligaments. A completely torn ligament not violating the synovial sheath does not allow dye filling. The roentgenogram provides poor circumstantial evidence.

Arthroscopy offers the only accurate method of assessing the status of the anterior cruciate ligament. It is possible to visualize the covering and the presence or absence of hemorrhage and to pull the tibia forward on the femur to observe the effect on the anterior cruciate ligament. Often the area of separation of attenuated old tears or acute tears can be seen by performing a drawer test during arthroscopy.

The so-called isolated anterior cruciate ligament tear has been the subject of debate by clinicians over the years, because prior to arthroscopy the joint could not be assessed to the extent that is possible now by anterior and posterior visualization. Such injury is considered isolated if there is no other abnormality that necessitates either arthroscopic treatment or arthrotomy. I have observed 16 patients in the past year who could be considered to have so-called isolated anterior cruciate ligament injury.

It is exceedingly rare in isolated cruciate ligament injury not to observe at least some hemorrhage in the wall of the posteromedial or posterolateral joint through posterior puncture; it is impossible to visualize this by anterior arthrotomy or anterior arthroscopy. The hemorrhage is frequently extrasynovial and involves the capsular tissues. Often hemorrhage disseminates to the posterior horn of the meniscus or the synovial attachment, yet there is no visible separation of the meniscus. Arthroscopic findings support the concept that when an injury is of such magnitude that it results in hemorrhagic change or tissue separation of the anterior cruciate ligament, there invariably is hemorrhage and tissue disruption in the capsular structures of the joint.

Eighteen of 113 patients examined in the past year who had anterior cruciate ligament injuries, either new or old, had degenerative changes of the joint or loose bodies from existing degeneration. Clinical instability was universally accompanied by the presence of a torn or attenuated anterior cruciate ligament; however, it should be noted that gross instability is not solely dependent on the presence or absence of the anterior cruciate ligament, but on the capsular supportive structures (e.g., the tibial collateral ligament on the medial side).

A torn anterior cruciate ligament accompanied or mimicked another condition in 25 of the 34 patients in our first series. At the time of examination, the ligaments were torn in such a way that they could not be repaired or the evaluation came at a time when absorption of the ligament did not render it repairable. It is important that a torn anterior cruciate ligament was not clinically recognized in many situations where it was seen arthroscopically. This supports the concept of early diagnosis in any suspected ligamentous injury, which is now possible by arthroscopy.

An accompanying meniscal injury is very common. In a second series of patients, seen from September 1975 to September 1976, meniscal injury accompanied anterior cruciate ligament tears in 49% of those examined under local or general anesthesia. This association should prompt awareness that when the preoperative diagnosis shows a torn meniscus, preparation should be made for necessary ligament repair or compensatory capsular reconstruction.

Of all patients in the two series, about half had extrasynovial and ligamentous injury and half had meniscal, patellar, or condylar disease.

The concomitant existence of cruciate ligament injury and degenerative arthritis, either suspected preoperatively or observed in patients with instability, points out the importance of the integrity of the anterior cruciate ligament. Many loose bodies that accompany this type of degenerative change can be observed only by posterior puncture. Articular loose bodies can be removed with the arthroscope, thus reducing morbidity without opening the compartment. In a few situations we have been able to arthroscopically remove large pieces of anterior cruciate ligament in either the posteromedial or posterolateral compartments, thus eliminating the need for arthrotomy.

The management of specific anterior cruciate ligament abnormalities is at the discretion and experience of the surgeon. Arthroscopy provides a definitive evaluation on which surgical judgment can be based.

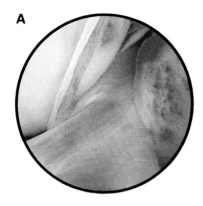

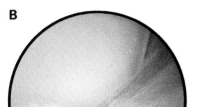

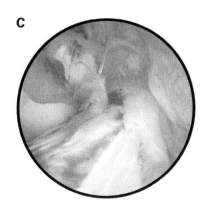

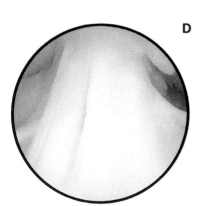

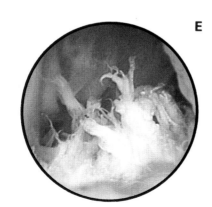

FIG. 12-1

A Torn anterior cruciate ligament does not show any gross separation. Hemorrhage appears to be subsynovial and interstitial. However, complete disruption of anterior cruciate ligament not evident from this view. Separate posterolateral puncture showed vast majority of cruciate ligament, which necessitated excision to remove symptoms.

B Common anterior cruciate ligament abnormality is extrusion of portion of ligament through slit in synovium. This eventually absorbs and rounds off. Small one asymptomatic.

C Complete disruption of anterior cruciate ligament, with fragment completely off pole.

D Longitudinal separations of cruciate ligament fibers, with loss of synovial covering and cabling of individual bundles, is sign of old partial tear in anterior cruciate ligament. Although ligament intact, instability demonstrates lack of ligament integrity

E Complete disruption of anterior cruciate ligament. Old complete disruption will show hemorrhage around it for up to 12 weeks following injury, but ligamentous tissue itself is avascular and contracted.

Tibial collateral

Arthroscopy provides an excellent means of evaluating a patient with tibial collateral ligament injury. Tenderness and pain over the tibial collateral area, increased by valgus stress, in the absence of palpable defect or marked instability, probably indicate an underlying torn meniscus. In the presence of hemorrhage, this diagnosis cannot be well established by arthography, but can be confirmed arthroscopically. Rapid rehabilitation therapy can be instituted if there is no instability or intra-articular lesion. Arthroscopy dictates appropriate early surgical intervention if there is internal derangement.

If the patient has a torn tibial collateral ligament and a palpable defect in that area, arthroscopic examination can discern any intra-articular abnormality that is amenable to surgery. If the lesion is well localized to the tibial collateral ligament off the femur and there is some instability, surgical exploration can be localized to that area and the repair carried out, resulting in rapid rehabilitation. An extensive arthrotomy is not necessary for joint exploration; it can be accomplished by arthroscopy.

Posterior cruciate

Isolated tears of the posterior cruciate ligament can be visualized by posteromedial puncture. It is not uncommon to see hemorrhage in that ligament without posterior instability. Isolated complete disruption of the posterior cruciate ligament can be confirmed at arthroscopy. I have seen two patients with complete absence of posterior cruciate ligament after injury and absorption.

Anteriorly, the view of the posterior cruciate ligament is blocked by the anterior cruciate ligament. However, in the total absence of this ligament, the posterior cruciate ligament is well defined and easily visualized anteriorly.

In the presence of both anterior and posterior cruciate ligament injury without complete detachment, marked subsynovial hemorrhage makes arthroscopic determination somewhat difficult from anterior puncture in the interondylar notch. Therefore, posteromedial inspection is essential in evaluating the status of the acutely injured posterior cruciate ligament in the absence of gross instability.

Lateral complex injury

The popliteus tendon can be visualized anterolaterally where it attaches to the femur. Avulsion of the tendon in that area has been identified. The normal course of the tendon is down through a sheath posterior and lateral to the meniscus. With anteromedial puncture, a small-diameter endoscope can be passed obliquely across the lateral compartment, and the popliteus tendon can be seen under and posterior to the meniscus (see Fig. 7-2).

Posterolateral inspection shows the popliteus tendon as it courses obliquely behind the meniscus. This area can house small loose bodies. In many instances the arthroscope can be introduced in this posterolateral sheath, and loose bodies can be vacuumed from the compartment. Disruption of the popliteus tendon along its course in the sheath has been visualized.

Arthroscopy has not been of particular value in diagnosing ruptures of the fibular collateral ligament and iliotibial band. They can be identified only by the presence of retrosynovial hemorrhage.

CHRONIC INSTABILITY

The evaluation of a patient with chronic instability of the joint can be enhanced by arthroscopy. The examination can clearly determine the extent of intra-articular abnormality and degenerative changes within the joint. Worn articular surfaces adversely affect the prognosis. The presence of retained menisci can be determined, and surgical management can be planned. The presence of an anterior cruciate ligament fronds caught in the joint can be identified and is amenable to arthrotomy at the time of reconstruction. Loose bodies can be removed through the arthroscopic cannulas.

There are some situations in which arthroscopic intra-articular inspection provides definitive information on which to further advise the patient of his problem, its surgical correction, and prognosis. When the arthroscopic inspection demonstrates no intra-articular abnormality that requires surgical intervention, the reconstructive procedure can proceed without the joint being entered.

The existence of retained posterior medial meniscal horns with partial cruciate ligament tear and degenerative arthritis is the most common instability problem that I have observed. Patients requiring reconstructive surgery can be accurately advised preoperatively of the surgical design. Often these patients have some apprehension because of multiple previous surgical procedures. Arthroscopy also can establish the presence or absence of torn menisci or abnormalities in the opposite compartment. If an existing lesion were unnoticed, prognosis would be hampered.

Chronic lateral instability of the anterolateral rotary type with lateral pivotal shifts is virtually nonexistent in the absence of the lateral meniscus. The mechanism of the lateral pivotal shift is dependent on the presence of a meniscus.

When a major problem is on the lateral side, arthroscopy not only establishes the status of that compartment but establishes the necessity for surgery on the medial compartment of the knee.

CYSTS

Baker's cysts are often associated with rheumatoid synovitis or chronic degenerative arthritis with loose bodies. Occasionally they are seen with a retained posterior horn with degenerative erosion of the posterior tibial condyle. The opening to the Baker's cyst may be visualized arthroscopically from the posteromedial compartment, and the inside of the cyst can be inspected. In some patients there is unidirectional flow of fluid from the joint to the Baker's cyst, as demonstrated by the placing of methylene blue in the joint. This dye flows into the Baker's cyst, but does not flow back to the posteromedial compartment. Debris of an articular nature has been seen within Baker's cysts. In cases where a Baker's cyst is secondary to another pathologic condition, correction of the condition will not eliminate the cyst. Resection of the cyst and removal of the articular debris are necessary for remission of symptoms.

Meniscal cysts are reported most commonly on the lateral side,[1] but I have seen several on the medial side. To save a patient unnecessary meniscectomy whenever possible, arthroscopy has been carried out. If there is no visible abnormality of the meniscus, the cystic mass is resected down to the meniscus. If the meniscus is not markedly degenerated at the entry site of the cyst, meniscectomy is not performed. However, a degenerative meniscus or considerable disruption of meniscal tissue with extension of the cyst to the meniscus warrants a meniscectomy. Presently I am following the progress of three patients who had resection of meniscal cysts without meniscectomy. One patient developed subsequent degenerative torn meniscus within 6 months; the other two patients have had no symptoms for a year.

Juxta-articular ganglion cysts can occur adjacent to the knee and mimic meniscal cysts. If arthroscopy demonstrates no intra-articular abnormality, the cyst is resected. Because these cysts do not track down to the menisci and go to the synovial paratendinous tissue, no arthrotomy or meniscectomy is necessary.

ANKYLOSIS

A few patients have developed ankylosis of the knee despite exhaustive physical therapy after previous multiple surgical procedures.

With the patients under general anesthesia, arthroscopy was performed to assess the interior of the joint and establish that there was no internal derangement causing the lack of motion. If no abnormality was found, the joint was manipulated and physical therapy was initiated, to the considerable benefit of the patient. It should be noted that arthroscopy provided confidence to both the physician and the patient that there was no offending intra-articular lesion and that surgical exploration and adhesiotomy were not necessary. Rehabilitation was relatively short.

OSGOOD-SCHLATTER DISEASE

A few patients with Osgood-Schlatter disease have had some referred knee complaints and an extra ossicle in the area of the tibial tubercle. With the patients under general anesthesia, arthroscopy was carried out to establish that no intra-articular abnormality existed. The extra ossicle of the tibial tubercle was excised, and rehabilitation therapy was instituted with absolute confidence that no underlying intraarticular abnormality went unnoticed.

PREOPERATIVE EVALUATIONS

Patients with gross disruption of ligamentous structures, whose knees are essentially disarticulated, do not require arthroscopic examination to assess the joint. Instillation of saline in the joint does not maintain distention, because of the capsular disruption.

There are patients with suspected or established ligamentous injuries in whom the presence or extent of the lesion is not easily established clinically. Such patients may have discomfort enough that they tighten the quadriceps muscle, making evaluation by x-ray examination and arthrogram difficult.

If hemarthrosis is present, arthrogram interpretation can be compromised. Hemarthrosis is not a contraindication to arthroscopy. The method that we have outlined of vacuuming the joint and instilling a 50-ml bolus of saline allows these joints to be inspected. It may be necessary to completely remove the blood and reinstill saline seven to ten times in order to cleanse the joint. Further, it might be necessary during viewing to instill saline under pressure from the syringe through the K-52 catheter and along the cannula to clear the area immediately in front of the viewing lens. It would be an unusual situation in which persistence did not result in an adequate and comprehensive evaluation.

REFERENCE

1. Becton, J. L., and Young, H. H.: Cysts of the semilunar cartilage of the knee, Arch. Surg. **90**:708-712, 1965.

Chapter 13

Synovial disease

Rheumatoid arthritis
Degenerative arthritis
Pigmented villa nodular synovitis
Osteochondromatosis
Gout
Pseudogout
Reiter's syndrome
Hemangioma
Psoriatic arthritis
Hemorrhagic synovium
Foreign bodies
Pedunculated nodular synovitis
Infection
Postoperative evaluations

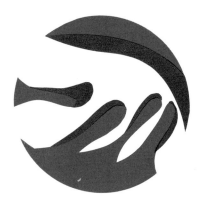

Arthroscopy provides easy access for direct visualization of the morphologic characteristics of the synovium. The suprapatellar pouch has the most abundant synovial surfaces for visualization. It may be possible with more experience to characterize the various rheumatologic conditions by their arthroscopic synovial morphology.

A number of patients have undergone diagnostic evaluations by arthroscopy for synovial disease in which the cause was not clear and the extent of the disease was not established. It has been possible to biopsy the synovium, either with direct vision or blindly when the condition is diffuse. Synovial fluid evacuated from the joint is useful for cell-block examination, which may show sheets of synovial tissue or articular debris, and tissue diagnosis (see Fig. 8-2).

RHEUMATOID ARTHRITIS

Rheumatoid arthritis is a protean condition. We have examined patients with negative results on serum tests and relatively low sedimentation rates, but whose histories suggested rheumatoid arthritis. Arthroscopy has been of benefit in establishing the diagnosis. With an established diagnosis, arthroscopy serves to follow the progress of medical treatment or to establish the extent of the articular damage.

Rheumatoid arthritis is characterized by long, fingerlike, projective villi with rounded ends, with a single blood vessel tracking up each villus. The surface area of these villi is incredible. The tips of the villi frequently have fibrinoid exudate (Fig. 13-1, *A*), which can be selectively stained with methylene blue. The wall has an extremely prominent vascular pattern of linear blood vessels, which accounts for the erythema accompanying this condition. There is considerable cloudiness in the joint when first entered, and cleansing of synovial fluid is essential for good visualization. Often a tuft of synovium is caught in the joint, usually between the patella and the femur, and becomes hemorrhagic.

Arthroscopy has been utilized to inspect the joints of patients who have had synovectomies. It is not unusual, in spite of excellent medical management, to see regrowth of synovium of a similar type as early as 6 months following knee-joint synovectomy, but the villi are smaller and more fibrotic.

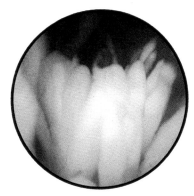

FIG. 13-1. Rheumatoid arthritis shows many fingerlike projections with fibrinoid tissue at tips, which can be selectively stained with methylene blue, and marked vascularity.

DEGENERATIVE ARTHRITIS

In degenerative arthritis the villi are rather fine and fibrinated. They are multiple, diffuse, shorter, and less round than those in rheumatoid arthritis (Fig. 13-2). This type of change is most common when there are loose bodies free in the joint. In some patients loose bodies have been engulfed so extensively throughout the synovium (see Fig. 8-2) that a synovectomy was required to ablate the offending foreign body from the articular surfaces. Early arthroscopic removal of loose bodies precludes this progressive synovitis.

Another form of degenerative arthritis is an acute inflammatory nonarticular arthritis. The patient may have a degenerative meniscus and perhaps mild tibia vara with degenerative compartment changes. Acutely inflamed joints appear the same as infected joints (Fig. 13-3). The presence of loose bodies can be established arthroscopically. They can be vacuumed from the joint, reversing the process.

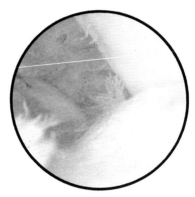

FIG. 13-2. Posterolateral compartment with marked proliferative villous synovitis seen in chronic degenerative changes, usually in presence of loose bodies.

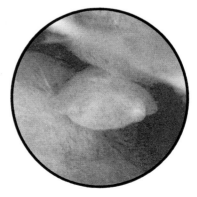

FIG. 13-3. Acute inflammation of joint, whether septic or due to degenerative changes, has extremely vascular synovium but without many villae.

PIGMENTED VILLA NODULAR SYNOVITIS

Pigmented villa nodular synovitis (Fig. 13-4) has been observed with surprising frequency. It was suspected in one patient, but in others degenerative arthritis was diagnosed. Arthroscopic findings are classic and descriptive. Although there are no articular changes in the early stages, long-standing pigmented villa nodular synovitis is accompanied by loss of articular tissue. With arthroscopy, invasion of the articular cartilage can be determined. The patient can be advised of the possibility of recurrence and the existence of degenerative changes that will affect the prognosis.

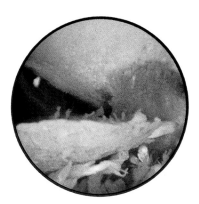

FIG. 13-4. Pigmented villa nodular synovitis with marked color changes within synovium and loss of articular surfaces in long-standing cases.

OSTEOCHONDROMATOSIS

Osteochondromatosis has been observed in three patients. In one, the nidus of the metaplasia was easily identified in the suprapatellar pouch and around the fat pad. It was especially important that there were multiple loose bodies in the posterolateral compartment. Because the thigh usually rests in external rotation, gravity carries the loose bodies to the posterolateral compartment. Also, the posterolateral and posteromedial compartments had areas of metaplasia. It was recommended to the referring surgeon that synovectomy be carried out, but also that the posteromedial and posterolateral compartments be opened to excise the areas of metaplasia to avoid recurrence.

Two patients had virtually hundreds of small osteochondromatose loose bodies. No metaplasia was observed in the synovium of the other compartments. For that reason, the joints were not opened, but all loose bodies were vacuumed from the joints with large cannulas. Histologic section identified these as osteochondromatoses. Because no metaplasia was identified in the synovium and in the absence of articular disease, no arthrotomy was carried out. Both patients have remained asymptomatic for over a year.

It is interesting to note that these multiple loose bodies differ from those of diffuse degenerative arthritis. In osteochondromatosis, loose bodies are not absorbed by the synovium. The synovial metaplastic areas have a budding appearance and shed the loose bodies rather than engulf them.

GOUT

Acute gouty arthritis can exist in the absence of an elevated uric acid level or family history of the disease. There may be acute nonarticular arthritis of a knee joint. Arthroscopic findings are classic,[1] including marked inflammation and considerable villi proliferations. Tophaceous gouty deposits within the villi appear very much like crystals and are highlighted by the light on the arthroscope; the eye is attracted to these deposits, and diagnosis is easily made. Confirmation can be made by direct-vision biopsy and histologic inspection or polarized-light arthroscopic identification.

PSEUDOGOUT

Pseudogout has been observed in two patients (Fig. 13-5). The calcium pyophosphate crystals are deposited in plaques, as opposed to the more isolated crystals seen in acute gout. The synovium is quite inflammed adjacent to the plaques. Direct biopsy provides material for polarized-light diagnosis. Biopsy can also be performed. Lavage of the joint at the time of arthroscopy is more than adequate treatment for a rather dramatic response.

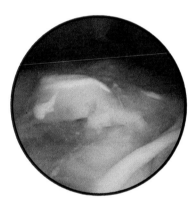

FIG. 13-5. Pseudogout shows calcium pyrophosphate crystals and plaques throughout synovial tissue. Vacuuming of joint and irrigation provide visual and pathologic diagnosis. Biopsy can be done with direct visualization to histologically establish diagnosis by polarized light on crystals.

REITER'S SYNDROME

Reiter's syndrome has been observed in one patient with an acutely inflammed joint in which the mucosa appeared very much like that seen in streptococcal infections. There were no articular changes in the joint and no villi. The joint had virtually hundreds of pieces of fibrinoid exudate, which were selectively stained with methylene blue for identification and confirmed by histologic section. Vacuuming out of these fibrinoid exudates resolved the synovitis sooner than would have been expected from the natural history of the condition.

HEMANGIOMA

Hemangioma was seen in a 19-year-old boy who had had multiple undiagnosed hemorrhages in his knee over time. Arthroscopic examination showed a synovial lining very much like that seen in pigmented villa nodular synovitis. Suprapatellar pouch inspection showed a large mass of hemangiomatous tissue with considerable fibrous bands. There was not much reactive synovitis except for the pigmented villi. Resection of the hemangioma rendered the patient asymptomatic.

PSORIATIC ARTHRITIS

Psoriatic arthritis (Fig. 13-6) has a very unique morphologic pattern. There is a marked arboretum of villi, which appear very lacy. Considerable vascular budding is seen within the wall of the synovium as well as in the arboretum of the tissue. Debris in the joint of a fibrinoid nature, but very shaggy, appearing like seaweed. It selectively stains with methylene blue. In contrast in rheumatoid arthritis the fibrinoid exudate is on the tips of the villi, giving a dumbbell appearance. In Reiter's syndrome, these loose bodies are rather round and flat.

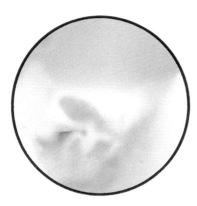

FIG. 13-6. Psoriatic arthritis shows lacelike villi and vascular budding within synovium.

HEMORRHAGIC SYNOVIUM

In any arthroscopic examination, attention should be paid to synovial hemorrhage (Fig. 13-7), especially in the area of the fat pad. This is usually indicative of a torn anterior cruciate ligament or an acute dislocation of the patella. On occasion, hemorrhagic synovium has been seen with contusion or parapatellar synovitis. In the latter condition, a shaggy fringe-type material about the patella catches between the patellofemoral junction, resulting in hemorrhage. Hemorrhage of pedunculated synovium has been seen in rheumatoid arthritis. Acute hemorrhage has a different characteristic and is easily identified morphologically.

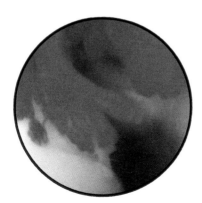

FIG. 13-7. Subsynovial hemorrhage will disseminate into villae. If in fat pad, usually indicates tear of anterior cruciate ligament. Acute dislocation of patella will show subsynovial hemorrhage as well.

FOREIGN BODIES

Persistent synovitis has been seen in some patients after penetration of the knee by an object (e.g., pieces of wood or nonradiopaque matter). With arthroscopy, injury or abrasion can be visualized in the joint and foreign bodies engulfed in the synovium can be identified. Local synovectomy is the treatment of choice.

PEDUNCULATED NODULAR SYNOVITIS

Several patients have had palpable loose bodies in the knee. Arthroscopy showed pedunculated nodular synovitis, which was corrected arthroscopically. There has been no recurrence in these patients.

INFECTION

Some patients have had acute knee infection in which the synovium appeared identical to that seen in streptococcal mucosal infection. Cultures showed positive findings, and in one patient the infection was indeed due to *Streptococcus*. We have not seen acute gonococcal arthritis arthroscopically.

POSTOPERATIVE EVALUATIONS

Inspection of the joint in patients who have had total knee replacement has not been particularly fruitful. We have documented photographically the regrowth of synovium in a patient who had had a geometric total-knee prosthesis for 18 months. She had catching and popping between the condylar surfaces, which was easily identifiable arthroscopically with active and passive motion. Injection of cortisone into the joint has rendered the patient asymptomatic for 2 years.

Some patients with Waldeus total-knee prostheses have been seen because they had pain. Due to the very tight fibrotic sac, examination is difficult, and it has not been possible to tell whether there was cement loosening; therefore, arthroscopy was not of much benefit.

I have been particularly hesitant in recommending that arthroscopy be performed routinely in patients with total-knee prostheses, because of the risk of infection. One patient with a suspected low-grade infection had loosening of a Waldeus prosthesis. During arthroscopy, hemarthrosis developed, resulting in acute exacerbation of the subclinical infection. Arthrotomy and drainage were necessary. The prosthesis was subsequently removed.

REFERENCE

1. O'Connor, R. L.: The role of arthroscopy in the management of crystal synovitis, J. Bone Joint Surg. **56**:206, 1974.

Index

154